Monetizing Misery: From Catastrophe to Cover-Up

Greg Wyatt

Monetizing Misery: From Catastrophe to Cover-Up

Copyright © 2024 by Greg Wyatt. All rights reserved.

All rights reserved. This book or any portion thereof may not be reproduced or used in any manner whatsoever without the express written permission of the publisher except for the use of brief quotations in a book review.

ISBN: 9798335418751

Editor and Interior Layout Design: Amy Sheesh

Cover Designer: Suzanne Daley

Every attempt has been made to source properly all quotes.

Printed in the United States of America

First Edition

GregWyatt.com

I dedicate this book to the memory of my children who are vaccine injured from their childhood immunizations and the millions of others who have suffered from the same fate.

"I know of nothing more despicable and pathetic than a man who devotes all the hours of the waking day to the making of money for money's sake."

John D. Rockefeller

(And yet, that is what people who monetize misery do. They spend all their time trying to part people from their money for a good cause. Inside this book, the illusion gets shattered.)

Disclaimer

Please note that the information provided herein comprises a compilation of evidence alongside personal opinions. These opinions are derived from factual information publicly accessible. It is important to emphasize that the intention is not to assert an all-encompassing or objective truth but to offer a perspective shaped by the available evidence.

Readers are strongly encouraged to conduct their own comprehensive research and exploration by following the links provided within this document. Each individual is responsible for delving into the subject matter independently, intending to evaluate whether their conclusions align with the assessment and analysis presented here.

This document serves as a foundational stepping stone toward a broader landscape of research and thorough inquiry. Exercising one's own discernment while also engaging in diligent fact-checking is paramount. Corrections and clarifications are welcome and encouraged.

Please approach this document as a springboard for deeper investigation and as an initial guide in pursuing knowledge. Your active participation in critical examination is essential to forming well-rounded conclusions.

The Purpose of This Book

The purpose of this book is not to malign or slander the individuals mentioned within its pages. Instead, it serves as a truthful account, with God as my witness, of my experiences. Initially, I believed I was on a Divine mission to change the world. However, as I became more involved, my intuition and intelligence revealed that things were not as they seemed.

Even more disheartening was the inability of those who idolized these figures to recognize the truth. This book is my gift of Truth to those who diligently seek it. Over eight years, I devoted thousands of hours to documenting my experiences. I knew that without such documentation, the truth would fade, allowing those responsible for what I consider the largest holocaust in human history to walk away as heroes when, in reality, they were anything but.

Contents

Disclaimer 7
The Purpose of This Book 8
Foreword 27
Introduction: 31
Exposing the Depths of Darkness 31
Chapter 1 35
The Harbinger of Change 35
Chapter 2 39
Setting the Scene: 39
Excited for the VaxXed Bus 39
Chapter 3 43
Jumping on the Black Bus 43
SECTION 1 45
Making an Example Out of 45
Del Bigtree 45
Chapter 4 47
Meeting Del 47
Chapter 5 51
Family Showmanship 51
   EXCLUSIVE EXPOSE: 51
   DEL BIGTREE'S FAMILY SECRETS 51
   A LEGACY OF SHOWMEN 51
   INTRIGUE BEYOND BLOODLINES 53
   TWO WORDS, ONE MYSTERY 54
   UNRAVELING THE ENIGMA 54

Chapter 6 57
A Tinseltown Tale of Chiefs and Silver Screens 57
   A SHOWBIZ PUZZLE: LOST TRUTHS AND
   AGENDAS... 57
   A TANGLED LEGACY OF LOVE AND LIES.......... 58
   THE CURTAIN CALL: THE MYSTIQUE CRUMBLES
   59
Chapter 7 63
Del's Father: Who is the Real Jack Groverland?..... 63
   FROM ARNEBOLD TO GROVERLAND 63
   FRITZ ARNEBOLD: A GLIMPSE INTO JACK'S
   FAMILY... 63
   THE CLOUDED ESCAPE: JACK'S BOLD
   JAILBREAK 64
   FROM MINISTER TO WORDSMITH 64
Chapter 8 67
Del's Wife: Lee Collette Nestor................................. 67
   LEE'S ANCESTRAL LINE 67
   PEGGY'S CREATIVE INFLUENCE........................ 67
Chapter 9 71
The Kennedy Connection 71
   OLEG CASSINI 71
   IGOR CASSINI INDICTED 73
   FROM ARISTOCRACY TO STARDOM.................. 73
   FALL FROM GRACE: A FAMILY AFFAIR 74
Chapter 10 77
Exposing Del Bigtree.. 77

   FROM STEAMY PRODUCTIONS TO PRODUCERS' GUILD 77

   TELEVISION STINTS AND TANGLED VISION 78

   FROM HOLLYWOOD TO VACCINE CONTROVERSY 78

   PURPLE THREADS 79

Chapter 11 81

Del Bigtree: A Wolf in Sheep's Clothing 81

   THE SUPREME COURT'S STANCE ON VACCINES 81

   BIGTREE'S CONTRADICTORY STANCE 81

   THE ILLUSION OF SAFETY AND COMPULSION . 82

   PERSONAL AUTONOMY AND CHOICE 82

   A PRO-VACCINE WOLF IN SHEEP'S CLOTHING . 82

SECTION 2 85

Divulging the "Game" 85

Chapter 12 87

Examining Tactics: Who are the Puppets and Provocateurs in the Web of Psuedo-Resistance? 87

   THE SHADOW PLAY OF DISSENT 87

   THE PUPPET THEATER 87

   A MIRAGE RESISTANCE 88

   ORCHESTRATED DISSENT IS THE SAFETY VALVE 88

   WHERE DECEPTION IS AN ART FORM 89

   CIRCULAR REPORTING 90

   THE ELUSIVE PUPPET MASTERS 91

   THE ILLUSION OF CHOICE 91

THE STRUGGLE FOR AUTHENTIC DISSENT 93
Chapter 13 95
A Quick Recap of How I Got Here 95
Chapter 14 103
How the Narrative is Manipulated 103
Chapter 15 105
Unraveling the Financial Schemes of the Health Freedom Movement 105
Chapter 16 107
Grifters - The Art of Deception 107
    COMMON TYPES OF GRIFTERS 107
    MOTIVATIONS OF GRIFTERS 108
    THE IMPACT OF GRIFTERS 108
    DETECTING AND PREVENTING GRIFTERS 109
    NOTICING THE BIGTREE GRIFT 110
Chapter 17 113
Familial Grifting – Passing Down Deception 113
    PASSING DOWN THE ART OF THE GRIFT 113
    EXAMPLES OF FAMILIAL GRIFTING CONTINUITY 114
    MOTIVATIONS BEHIND PASSING DOWN GRIFTING 114
    CONSEQUENCES OF PASSING DOWN DECEPTION 115
    MAKING CONNECTIONS 115
Chapter 18 117
MLM Millionaires: The Exploitative Structures of Multi-Level Marketing 117

UNDERSTANDING MULTI-LEVEL MARKETING 117

THE PYRAMID SCHEME RENAMED................. 118

EXPLOITING THE VULNERABLE...................... 118

VULTURES OF THE HEALTH FREEDOM
MOVEMENT 118

Chapter 19 121

The Zeolite Debate: Natural Benefits vs. Synthetic
Schemes 121

UNDERSTANDING ZEOLITES.......................... 121

THE RISE OF SYNTHETIC ZEOLITES AND TRS 122

TRS: A MULTI-LEVEL MARKETING SCHEME... 123

THE USUAL SUSPECTS.................................... 123

BLACK OXYGEN ORGANICS: 124

A CASE STUDY IN MLM FAILURE 124

Chapter 20 127

Controlled Opposition vs. Orchestrated Dissent and
Psuedo-Resistance: Manipulating Dissent for
Strategic Gains 127

PSEUDO-RESISTANCE IN THE "MEDICAL
FREEDOM" MOVEMENT 128

THE IMPACT OF ORCHESTRATED DISSENT ... 130

DETECTING AND COUNTERING PSUEDO-
RESISTANCE... 131

THE OVERLAP.. 132

Chapter 21 135

Charities and Fraudulent Promises - The Illusion of
Change 135

ILLUSION OF CHANGE.................................... 135

MOVEMENTS IN THE SPOTLIGHT: 136
THE CHARITABLE ILLUSION............................ 136

Chapter 22 139
How Dishonest People Appear Honest.................. 139
   CONFIDENCE AND CHARISMA 139
   DETAIL AND CONSISTENCY 139
   EMOTIONAL MANIPULATON 140
   BODY LANGUAGE AND MICRO-EXPRESSIONS 140
   REPUTATION AND SOCIAL PROOF 141
   SELECTIVE TRUTHS 141
   GENUINE EMOTIONS.. 142
   MIRRORING AND BUILDING RAPPORT 142
   DEFLECTION AND REDIRECTION 142
   PREPARATION AND PRACTICE 143

Chapter 23 145
The Struggle to Acknowledge Being Duped by an Organization 145
   COGNITIVE DISSONANCE................................. 145
   SUNK COST FALLACY 145
   IDENTITY AND EGO PROTECTION 146
   SOCIAL PRESSURE... 146
   HOPE AND OPTIMISM....................................... 146
   MISINFORMATION AND DENIAL 147

Chapter 24 149
Unmasking PsyOps - The Art of Psychological Operations 149
   WHAT ARE PSYCHOLOGICAL OPERATIONS? .. 149

    THE HISTORICAL ROOTS OF PSYOPS 149
    THE PSYCHOLOGICAL TOOLBOX 150
    COUNTERMEASURES AND RESILIENCE 151

Chapter 25 153
The Evolution of Psychological Operations 153
    THE ORIGINS OF PSYOPS 153
    WORLD WAR I AND WORLD WAR II 153
    THE COLD WAR ERA 154
    MODERN PSYOPS 154
    THE ROLE OF PSYOPS TODAY 155
    KEY PRINCIPLES OF PSYOPS 155

Chapter 26 157
Medical Psychological Operations (Medical PsyOps)
.... 157
    THE EMERGENCE OF MEDICAL PSYOPS 157
    PRINCIPLES OF MEDICAL PSYOPS 157
    MODERN APPLICATIONS 158
    ETHICAL CONSIDERATIONS 159

Chapter 27 161
Hollywood IS the Propaganda Machine 161
    CATCHING THE DISSENTERS 163
    THE ILLUSION OF ANTI-VACCINE OPPOSITION
.... 165
    SHEEPHERDERS LEADING THE FLOCK 166
    LIMITED HANGOUT OPERATION 166
    WHERE DOES BIGTREE FIT IN? 166

Chapter 28 169

The Art of Grifting – A Cynical Exploitation 169
    THE CON ARTIST'S SYMPHONY 169
    THE ENABLERS OF GRIFT 169
    THE TANGLED WEB OF DECEPTION 170
    MONETIZING MISINFORMATION 171
    THE CONSEQUENCES OF GRIFTING 171

Chapter 29 173

Non-Profits: The Manipulation of Social Good 173
    THE FAÇADE OF ALTRUISM 173
    CHARITY BEGINS (AND ENDS) AT THE TOP 173
    PUPPETEERS OF CHANGE 174
    THE MIRAGE OF SOCIAL SERVICES AND CHANGE 174
    UNMASKING THE CHARADE 175

Chapter 30 177

Billionaire "Philanthropists" and the Swaying of Medical Information: The Case of Bill and Melinda Gates 177
    THE GATES' ADVOCACY FOR VACCINES 177
    POPULATION CONTROL STATEMENTS 177
    LEGAL AND ETHICAL CONCERNS 178
    THEIR WORK OVERSEAS 178
    INFLUENCE ON MEDICAL INFORMATION 179

Chapter 31 181

Follow the Money – The Lucrative Pandemic-Fueled Windfall for Alleged 'Anti-Vaccination' Groups 181
    THE BIRTH OF ADVOCACY GROUPS 181

EYE-OPENING 2020 TAX RECORDS	182
Chapter 32	187
VaxXed Revisited	187
SECTION THREE:	191
Scientology in the Health Freedom Movement	191
Chapter 33	193
The Sinister Alliance: Scientology and the Health Freedom Movement	193
Chapter 34	197
The Digital Web: Decoding Internet Addresses and the Shadowy Connections	197
SECTION FOUR:	199
Why the Tactics Work	199
Chapter 35	201
The Struggle of Cognitive Dissonance	201
WHEN FOOD IS MORE THAN FUEL	201
THE UNSETTLING ENCOUNTER	201
CLASH OF BELIEFS	202
SEEKING RESOLUTION	202
Chapter 36	205
The Tightrope of Cognitive Dissonance	205
DEL BIGTREE'S MESSAGE: A FEARFUL SERENADE	205
DECEPTION IN THE ECHO CHAMBER	205
SECTION FIVE:	207
Other Players in the Monetizing Misery Drama	207
Chapter 37	209

The Canary Party's Betrayal and the Puppeteers Behind the Curtain 209
   ORIGINS OF DISTRUST 209
   BEGINNING WITH A COMPROMISED MISSION 210
   FRACTURES AND FALLOUT 211
   THE RESISTANCE 212

Chapter 38 215
Andrew Wakefield: The Quintessential pHARMa 'Martyr' 215
   CLARITY ON HIS ROLE 216
   THE SHOCKING NARRATIVE THAT GOT SWEPT UNDER THE RUG 217

Chapter 39 219
Collapsing Tragedy: The Untimely Death of Alex Spourdalakis 219
   DESPERATION AND FRUSTRATION 219
   DOCUMENTARY AND BROKEN PROMISES 220
   THE WAKEFIELD AND TOMMEY CONNECTION 220

Chapter 40 223
Capitalizing on Murder?: How Did They Miss the Warning Signs? 223
   BEFORE ALEX'S DEATH 223
   AFTER ALEXS DEATH: 224
   UNANSWERED QUESTIONS & LACK OF SCRUTINY 224
   ETHICAL IMPLICATIONS 224

Chapter 41 227

Exploiting Autism: The Dark Side of Polly Tommey and the Autism Trust 227

Chapter 42 229

The Mystery of Brandy Vaughan 229

Chapter 43 233

The Questionable Whistleblower: Brandy Vaughan's Timeline 233

    EARLY LIFE AND CAREER 233

    RETURN TO THE UNITED STATES AND ENTRY INTO THE ANTI-VACCINE MOVEMENT 234

        CONTEXT OF THE ANTI-VACCINE MOVEMENT 235

    ANALYSIS AND QUESTIONS 235

    THE AGGRESSIVE POSTHUMOUS HANDLER .. 237

    MY FINAL ANALYSIS 238

Chapter 44 239

One of the CIA's Thirteen Illuminati Families and Presidential Hopeful, RFK, Jr. 239

Chapter 45 243

RFK Jr. and Del Bigtree's FOIA Charade 243

Chapter 46 245

JB Handley and "Ending the Autism Epidemic" ... 245

    THE CONTROVERSIAL RECOMMENDATIONS . 245

    NO TRUE ALTERNATIVE 246

    THE INFLUENCE OF THE BLACK BUS TEAM .. 246

    THE SHIFT IN PERSPECTIVE 246

    A STAGNANT PERSPECTIVE 247

SECTION SIX: 249

Grifting Projects: What the Pseudo-Resistance Uses to Prey Upon the Masses 249

Chapter 47 251

SB277 - The Turning Point 251

SB277: A WATERSHED MOMENT IN IMMUNIZATION LEGISLATION 251

THE TIGHTENING OF VACCINE REQUIREMENTS 251

LEGACY PROVISIONS-THE GRANDFATHER CLAUSE 252

IMPLICATIONS AND IMPLEMENTATION 252

CONTINUED ADVOCACY AND ENGAGEMENT . 252

Chapter 48 255

SB277 - The Perfect Storm 255

HOW SB277 TURNED INTO AN OPPORTUNITY TO EXPLOIT 255

THE DISENFRANCHISED SEEK REPRESENTATION 255

EXPLOITING THE MOMENTUM 256

MOVIES, BOOKS, AND MONETIZING MISERY . 256

Chapter 49 259

The Autism Trust—What Are the Facts? 259

POLLY AND JONATHON TOMMEY 259

SHADY LAND DEAL? BERTHA & KEN BRADLEY 259

FROM ADULT ENTERTAINMENT TO AUTISM TRUST 260

ELABORATE PROMISES AND MASTER PLANS 261

SECTION SEVEN: 263

Medical Truths that Must Be Ignored for the "Game" to Work.. 263

Chapter 50 265

Rockefeller Medicine: A Nefarious Transformation from Oil to Pharmaceuticals................................. 265

    THE RISE OF ROCKEFELLER AND THE MONOPOLISTIC EMPIRE................................... 265

    AN OPPORTUNISTIC SHIFT TO MEDICINE........ 265

    THE FLEXNER REPORT: A STRATEGIC ELIMINATION OF COMPETITION...................... 266

    THE BIRTH OF PETROLEUM-BASED MEDICINE 266

    VACCINES: THE ULTIMATE PROFIT-DRIVEN PUBLIC HEALTH STRATEGY 267

    THE CONSEQUENCES OF ROCKEFELLER'S MEDICAL MONOPOLY.. 267

    THE DARK SIDE OF ROCKEFELLER MEDICINE 268

    THE ULTIMATE MOTIVE: MONETIZING MISERY 268

Chapter 51 269

Unveiling the Flaws of VAERS: An Exposé on Vaccine Surveillance... 269

    CREATION OF VAERS 269

    COLLABORATION AND OVERSIGHT 270

    CRITICISM AND CONTROVERSY...................... 270

Chapter 52 273

The Vaccine Injury Compensation Program: A Taxpayer-Funded Façade................................ 273

ORIGINS OF THE NCVIA 273
　　CREATION OF THE VICP 273
　　COLLABORATION AND OVERSIGHT 274
　　CRITICISM AND CONTROVERSY 274
Chapter 53 277
Barbara Loe Fisher 277
Chapter 54 281
The Harvard Study on Underreporting of Vaccine
Adverse Events 281
　　THE HARVARD STUDY 281
　　REASONS FOR UNDERREPORTING 281
　　INACCESSIBILITY OF COMPENSATION 282
Chapter 55 283
The Dark History of Fetal Cell Lines in Vaccines .. 283
　　THE ORIGIN OF FETAL CELL LINES 283
　　WI-38 AND MRC-5 283
　　HEK-293 284
　　WALVAX-2 AND OTHER CELL LINES 284
　　THE "WATER BAG" ABORTION METHOD 285
　　RESEARCH AND VACCINE DEVEOPMENT 285
　　THE ISSUE OF BLOODLINE MISMATCHES 285
　　ETHICAL AND MORAL CONCERNS 286
Chapter 56: 287
The Concerning Ingredients in Vaccines 287
　　ALUMINUM 287
　　FORMALDEHYDE 288
　　THIMEROSAL 288

POLYSRBATE 80 289
ANIMAL CELL LINES 289
ACETONE 289
E. COLI 290
YEAST 290
GLUTARALDEHYDE 290
THE ISSUE OF INJECTION 291
SIDE EFFECTS LISTED IN VACCINE INSERTS . 291
THE 13.1 WARNING 292

Chapter 57: 295
Uncovering SV40: The Simian Virus Presence in
Vaccines 295
   DISCOVERY AND ORIGIN 295
   HEALTH IMPLICATIONS 295
   PUBLIC AWARENESS AND ADVOCACY 296

Chapter 58 297
The Gap Between Informed Consent and Vaccine
Information Sheets 297
   UNDERSTANDING INFORMED CONSENT 297
   DISCREPANCIES IN VACCINE INFORMATION
   SHEETS 298
   CLOSING THE GAP 298

Chapter 59 301
Well-Child Visits: Vaccination Mandates and the
Erosion of Informed Consent 301
   WELL-CHILD VISITS HAVE BECOME VACCINE
   VISITS 301
   REFUSAL AND COERCION 301

INFORMED CONSENT AND THE RIGHT TO
REFUSE 302
LEGISLATIVE HURDLES AND MANDATORY
VACCINATION 302
PRESERVING INFORMED CONSENT AND
PARENTAL RIGHTS 302

Chapter 60 305
The Unseen Hand of Ignaz Semmelweis 305
INVISIBLE THREATS 305
REVELATION IN THE MORGUE 306
CONTAMINATED HANDS: AN UNSEEN MENACE
.... 306
THE SEMMELWEIS EFFECT 307
THE LEGACY OF SEMMELWEIS: LESSONS
UNLEARNED 307

Chapter 61 309
Terrain Theory Reigns Supreme 309
DUELING DOCTRINES: GERM VS. TERRAIN
THEORY 309
THE HEART OF TERRAIN THEORY 310

Chapter 62 313
The Hidden Code: Viruses Engraved in Our DNA . 313
VIRUSES EMBEDDED WITHIN 313
ARCHITECTS OF EVOLUTION: RETROVIRUSES
.... 314
SILENT INHABITANTS: DORMANT VIRUSES 314
FROM DORMANCY TO DANCE: CHICKEN POX 315
SHINGLES: THE VIRAL ENCORE 315

THE INNER TRIGGER: ENERGETIC ACTIVATION 315

Chapter 63 317

Measles Virus as a Cancer Protectorate 317

    THE MEASLES VIRUS: A HISTORICAL PERSPECTIVE 317

    ONCOLYTIC VIRUSES 317

    MEASLES VIRUS AND CANCER: A SURPRISING CONNECTION 318

    THE MECHANISM BEHIND THE ANTI-CANCER ACTION OF MEASLES 318

    CLINICAL TRIALS AND POTENTIAL APPLICATIONS 319

SECTION EIGHT: 321

My Contributions to the Fight 321

Chapter 64 323

Handing Out My "Are Vaccines Safe?" Truth Cards 323

    VACCINE INJURY MEMORIAL VEHICLE 327

Chapter 65 329

The Weaponization of Social Media: Censorship, Propaganda, and Controlling the Narrative 329

    THE RISE OF SOCIAL MEDIA CONTROL 330

    PANDEMIC PARADIGM: A PREFACE TO EXTREME CENSORSHIP 331

    "POLITICAL" SILENCING: THE TYRANNY OF "MAJORITY" OPINION—PERCEIVED OR REAL, WE'LL NEVER KNOW 333

    THE EASE OF PROPAGANDA DISSEMINATION 335

Chapter 66 339
Corporate Influence and Political Agendas 339
    FROM MYSPACE TO METAVERSE:
    CONSOLIDATING CONTROL 341
Chapter 67 343
The Intersection of Big Tech and Big Pharma 343
Epilogue: 347
A Call to Awareness and Action 347
A Letter from a Parent: 349
References 351
About the Author—Greg Wyatt 353

Foreword

In the shadowed corridors of modern history, a pivotal moment emerged on April 1, 2016, when the world witnessed the unveiling of a cinematic revelation: "VaxXed: From Cover-Up to Catastrophe (2016)." A beacon of hope emerged for the anguished hearts of parents grappling with the profound consequences of their children's vaccination journeys, a labyrinth fraught with chemical pitfalls.

It was a day etched in my memory that marked the beginning of an extraordinary odyssey. I found myself among those resilient souls who dared to challenge the norms, question the established order, and demand the truth concealed beneath layers of misinformation. Yes, I was one of those parents, a father who cradled two innocent souls, Weston and Emily, both casualties in a battle against the very rites meant to protect them.

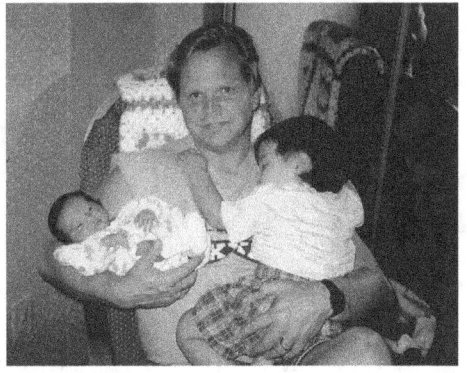

In the early dawn of 2013, a digital lifeline drew me into a realm of shared grief and unwavering determination. The labyrinthine networks of social media, pulsating with the heartbeat of virtual communities, became my haven. The symphony of heartrending narratives swelled on platforms like Facebook and YouTube, a crescendo of voices recounting tragedies that had befallen their cherished progeny.

Monetizing Misery

Yet, amidst this chorus of despair, a stark truth emerged—a revelation that rattled the very foundations of my understanding. A staggering 90% of those who bared their souls in this digital tapestry were single mothers, left abandoned by partners, forsaken by institutions, and cast adrift in the tempest of their children's afflictions. The statistics painted a grim tableau of shattered dreams and solitary struggles, where mothers stood as fierce sentinels, resolute in their battles for justice.

A year unfurled its wings, and with it, the seed of a fervent resolve took root within me. I unfurled a banner of public awareness, birthing "The Vaccine Truth Movement," an entity through which I sought to transmute my anguish into a weapon of mass

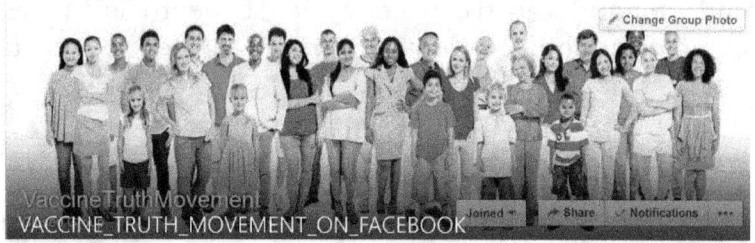

enlightenment. The torrent of messages that inundated my digital sanctum was a testament to shared pain and a clarion call to action. Daily, a litany of kindred spirits reached out, their stories interwoven with mine in despair and, ultimately, defiance.

I embarked on an unforeseen path that led me to relinquish the allure of early retirement, a decision that marked the beginning of a vocation born from adversity. The landscape of my endeavors was cast across the digital expanse, where Facebook groups sprang forth like constellations, and a grassroots movement was choreographed to traverse the tapestry of the United States, leapfrogging borders to whisper across the globe.

Once a solitary whisper, my voice found resonance on the airwaves of countless virtual broadcasts. The tale of my children, the heartrending chronicle of their affliction, reverberated through the digital ethers, a siren call to those who would listen. The world bore witness as my modest undertaking, "The Vaccine Truth Movement," erupted into an inferno, a beacon that ignited minds and catalyzed action. But the tale that unfolded was far from the idyllic symphony of change and camaraderie I had envisaged.

The veil of naiveté lifted, unraveling illusions as swiftly as they had been spun. The corridors of power, it seemed, were not as they appeared—shadows danced behind the scenes, and questions unfurled like banners in the wind. A year into this consuming journey, a gnawing realization took root. Doubt sprouted like an insidious vine, wrapping its tendrils around my once-unwavering conviction. As the threads of skepticism wove through my consciousness, I was compelled to peer beyond the veneer to probe the depths of the enigma "VaxXed."

This dear reader, is the overture of my encounter with the puppeteers who orchestrated the spectacle, the architects of the movie that was meant to be a rallying cry yet held secrets darker than the night itself. The following chapters will unfurl the tapestry of my dealings with those who stood behind the celluloid curtain—a story of intrigue, revelation, and a quest for truth that would spiral into the uncharted abyss of human ambition.

Monetizing Misery

Introduction:

Exposing the Depths of Darkness

As I began writing my book, *Light in the Darkness*, I was confronted with the sobering realization that specific topics demanded more than mere chapters within a single book. The sprawling grip of eugenics, vaccine damage, and the Health Freedom Movement warranted separate narratives to unravel their complexities without overshadowing the poignant tale of my father's struggle.

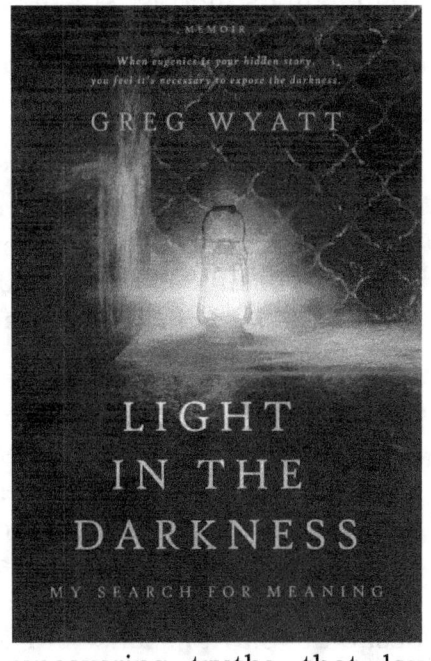

My proficiency in research, honed in an era of card catalogs and dusty archives, proved invaluable in uncovering truths that lay obscured beneath layers of obfuscation. Yet, my journey into the perilous realms of vaccine injury and eugenics began not as an academic pursuit but as a profoundly personal odyssey catalyzed by the anguish of witnessing my own children's descent into severe autism, their innocence marred by the toxicity of vaccines.

The failure to foresee the dangers of vaccination before it touched my family remains a burden I bear with profound remorse. Determined to spare others from a similar fate, I embarked on a crusade to disseminate knowledge unencumbered by the allure of monetary gain. Despite the immense toll exacted on every facet of my being—financially, emotionally, physically, mentally, and spiritually—I refused to commodify suffering, steadfast in my commitment to illuminate the shadows cast by modern medicine.

The revelation of my origins, entangled in the web of eugenics, further fueled my quest for understanding. Learning of my conception as a product of state-sponsored sterilization and selective breeding under the guise of "superior stock" ignited a fervent pursuit of biological siblings and deeper insights into the insidious practices of eugenics.

The diagnosis of severe autism in my children thrust me into a battle against a medical establishment more concerned with managing symptoms than unraveling the mysteries of causation. Faced with dismissive attitudes and an absence of support, I turned to the education system, only to be met with resistance and accusations of fraud—a desperate ploy to silence our advocacy.

This book is a testament to resilience, a defiant proclamation of vindication in adversity. It lays bare the scars of a life marred by injustice and betrayal, a chronicle of battles waged, and victories won, each page a testament to the indomitable spirit of a mother driven by love and righteous indignation.

In the tumultuous landscape of the Health Freedom movement, I have stood as a sentinel against the exploitation of suffering, refusing to yield to the temptation of profiteering. While I refrain from naming every malefactor that festers within its ranks, I offer a guide to discerning their machinations, a roadmap to navigating the treacherous waters of deceit and duplicity.

For those who dare to confront the darkness that lurks beneath the veneer of progress, this book serves as a beacon of hope—a rallying cry for justice and the unyielding pursuit of truth.

Chapter 1

The Harbinger of Change

The cusp of spring in 2011 heralded a parcel, innocuous in appearance yet laden with the weight of destiny. As I gingerly unfurled its contents, the revelation unfurled before me—an anthology of ink and parchment, a complex narrative stitched together with the meticulous care of a war strategist marshaling troops for a covert battle. Thousands of sheets bore the arcane script of medical records, a testament to 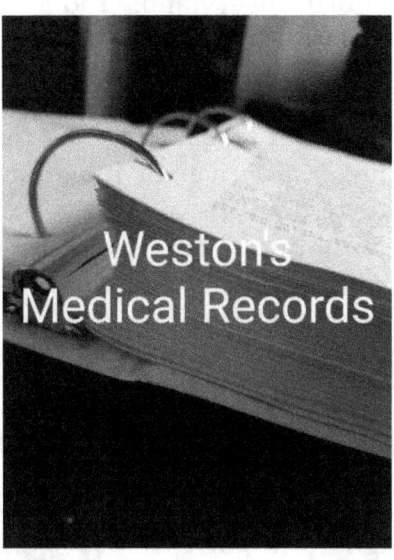 the journey my son had undertaken from his nascent days through the tender arc of his third year, spanning the years 1998 to 2001.

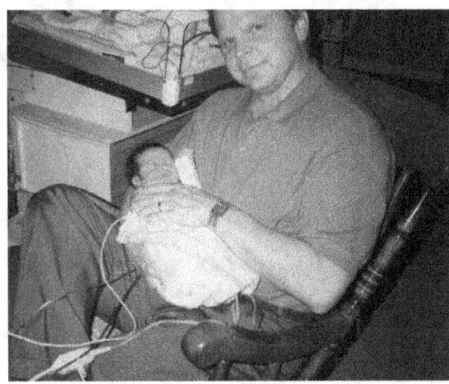 The sender, none other than the United States federal government, had unwittingly thrust me into the heart of a mystery—a puzzle I was compelled to decipher. The pages

chronicled a symphony of visits to the citadel of pediatric care, Ponderosa Pediatrics, where my son, once a paragon of health, had embarked on a harrowing odyssey. The innocuous well-baby appointments, once a ritual of growth and safeguarding, had birthed a specter of sickness that consumed him relentlessly. Their answer, a cyclical chorus of Tylenol and Motrin, fell as hollow notes against the cacophony of questions that reverberated within us.

The passage of time slipped through our fingers, a river of moments that bore us inexorably toward an irreversible precipice. By 2001, the somber pronouncement had been cast—autism, a shadow cast over my son's once-untouched horizon. The chasm between the boy who once embodied perfection, and the one now ensnared by a condition we had not invited, was an abyss into which we stumbled, ignorant of the forces that had conspired against us.

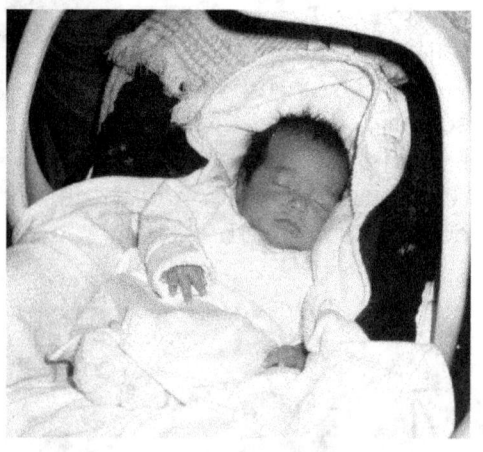

A fervent ember ignited within me, fueled by an unquenchable desire to forge a world where the shadows of affliction would never shroud the innocent laughter of children, where the echoes of anguish would fade into oblivion, and where the tapestry of my cherished family would remain unblemished by the horrors that fate had wrought upon us.

In the hushed corridors of uncertainty, as the tendrils of comprehension reached out, I found myself irrevocably bound to a mission—to unearth the truth concealed beneath layers of ambiguity, to shine a light upon the path we had unwittingly traversed, and to sound a clarion call that would resonate through the annals of time. This is the chronicle of my metamorphosis, the genesis of a journey that would lead me to confront the very fabric of existence, unraveling the tapestry of secrets woven into the narrative of my son's life—a narrative that was forever altered by those seemingly innocuous well-baby visits, each a harbinger of profound change.

Chapter 2

Setting the Scene:

Excited for the VaxXed Bus

In the monumental year of 2016, visionary creators, filmmakers, editors, and photographers, coalesced into an unstoppable force—the vanguard of change, the architects of a movement. Their masterpiece, "VaxXed," a clarion call that reverberated through the annals of time, set the stage for a chapter that would eclipse even the most audacious of dreams.

Enter the stage, the resplendent "VaxXed Nation Tour," a phenomenon that swept across the canvas of the United States, igniting hearts and minds as it traced a path through the heartlands and bustling cities alike. It was not a mere journey—it was a pilgrimage of purpose, woven with intention, each stop 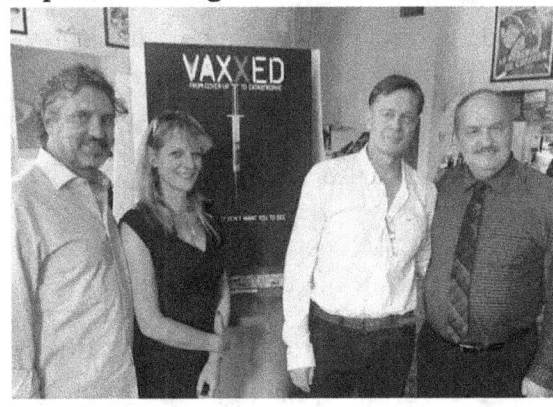 strategically selected to intersect with the corridors of power, where members of the United States House Committee of Oversight & Government Reform held sway over the institution that is the CDC.

The bus tour was more than just a physical movement; it was a force of transformation, a journey of advocacy and enlightenment that crackled with electric vitality. At each destination, the silver screen would unfold, casting its incandescent glow upon screens that had become the canvas of change. Screenings were more than mere spectacles—they were rallying cries, opportunities for interaction, for the exchange of truths, and for the liberation of voices long stifled. People who called themselves "truthers" and "medical freedom advocates" flocked to enjoy the events and pose for pictures with the faces of the movement. I was no different, intoxicated by the rallying cry to unite against the nefarious agendas and powers that be. For once, it seemed like something would be accomplished.

As the wheels of the VaxXed Nation bus rolled ceaselessly, stories intertwined, converging and diverging like tributaries feeding into a river of revelation. Autism families, health professionals, and the silent warriors of vaccine injury—each voice found its chorus, harmonizing in a crescendo of raw emotion. Q&A sessions echoed with the resonance of newfound understanding, building bridges between hearts and minds that had once stood estranged.

Numbers amassed, not as mere statistics, but as tributes to human resilience, resolve, and the indomitable spirit of those who dared to shatter the shackles of silence. Almost 1000 stories, meticulously captured on film, brought to life a mosaic of suffering, strength, and solidarity. And beyond the silver screen, on the digital tapestry of VaxXed.com, 6,900 written narratives bore witness to the global symphony of pain and perseverance.

A towering crescendo climaxed in the whispered names, a collective memorial etched upon the bus—a tapestry of remembrance that bore witness to those who had been felled by the very instruments of health they had sought. Names of the injured, names of the fallen, each one a chapter in a narrative that galvanized action, inspired unity, and underscored the solemn purpose of the journey.

And so, against the backdrop of the VaxXed Nation bus, against the walls of stories, statistics, and steadfast resolve, a movement unfurled—an anthem of health freedom, an iridescent symbol of tenacity, and a testament to the power of voices united. The chapters ahead would chronicle not just a tour, but a transformation—a movement that shook the very foundations of complacency and sowed the seeds of change in the fertile soil of collective consciousness.

Chapter 3

Jumping on the Black Bus

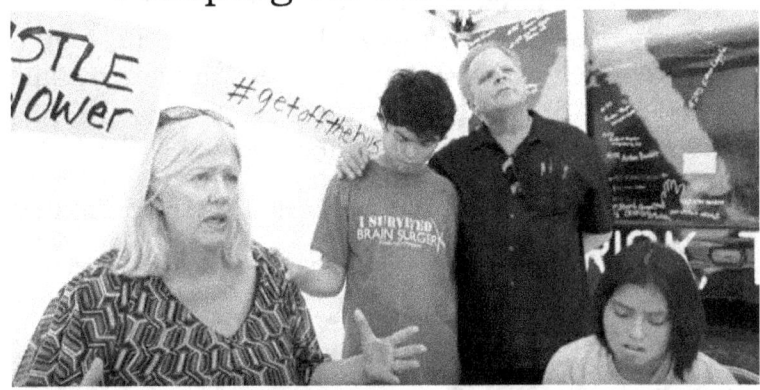

Del Bigtree rapidly ascended to the echelons of American iconhood, courtesy of his groundbreaking documentary "VaxXed." His influence extended to parents of vaccine-afflicted children and encompassed me—a father beset by the ordeal of two vaccine-injured offspring.

In the shadows of time, parents united within grassroots groups, their hearts aflame with the aspiration for transformative change. This collective effort spanned years, fueled by the fervent hope of sculpting a new reality.

Yet, a seismic shift altered the landscape on that fateful April 1st, 2016. The unveiling of Del Bigtree's magnum opus, "VaxXed," reverberated across the nation, kindling flames of awareness in the hearts of parents and in my own. A pair of vaccine-injured children bore testimony to the urgency of the cause, propelling me toward my inevitable calling.

With the dawn of the following month, a newfound energy took shape—a black bus emblazoned with purpose embarked on a nationwide journey, a VaxXed tour igniting the flames of consciousness and financial support in equal measure. Each autistic, handicapped, and chemically injured individual was invited to sign the bus and was assigned a corresponding number.

The cadence of fate beckoned my attention as whispers of their impending visit to Arizona reached my ears— a strategic pit stop in 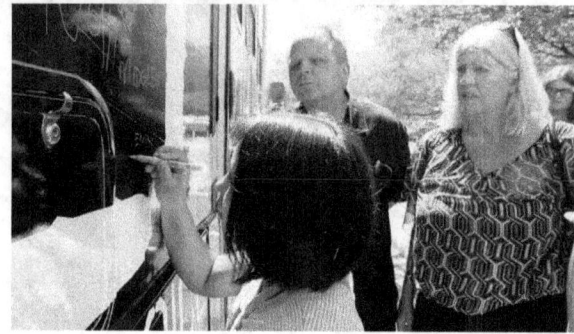 congressional districts that harbored the power to reshape laws. This juncture became a convergence of destiny, an opportunity to bridge the gap between spectatorship and active participation, as I set my sights on extending a helping hand.

The stage was set at the Paradise Valley Community Center—an arena for transformation, where intentions merged, alliances solidified, and narratives were 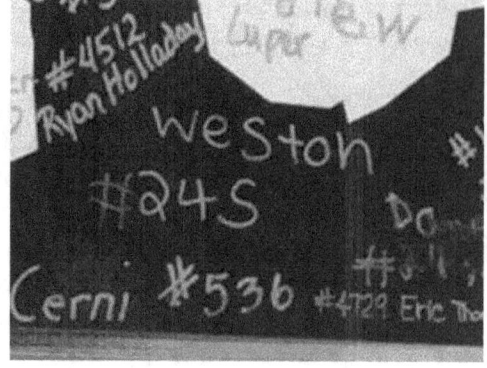 poised to be rewritten.

SECTION 1

Making an Example Out of Del Bigtree

Chapter 4

Meeting Del

For nearly seven decades, my life has been dedicated to pursuing knowledge. Since my boyhood, an insatiable curiosity drove me to delve beneath the surface, questioning the very fabric of our existence. The mysteries of the azure sky, the enigma of Earth's brown hues, and the intricate dance of human behaviors consumed my thoughts.

However, amidst my intellectual journey, a singular figure emerged on my radar, captivating my attention in ways I never anticipated. Del Matthew Bigtree, the perplexing leader of the anti-vaccine movement, became an irresistible puzzle that refused to release its grip on my mind despite my earnest attempts to resist.

The community center's auditorium sprawled before us, a sizable expanse teeming with potential. Joyce, Emily, and I embarked on our journey, arriving a good half-hour before the clock struck 1:00 p.m.

Navigating the unfamiliar terrain, we trod cautiously, exchanging glances as we found our seats. A friendly face welcomed us at the door, setting the tone for what was to come.

The room was a puzzle of faces—some undoubtedly parents, while others remained a mystery. With discerning eyes, we assessed the assembly, realizing that most of those present were not part of our shared journey but a new wave of future parents and supporters of the movement, significant in their own way to the advancement of the cause.

Amidst this sea of unfamiliarity, there were people that recognized me, a testament to the reach of my efforts. Familiar faces emerged from the crowd, seeking connection, their outstretched hands a testament to the impact of my work. The echoes of my reception at the CDC resurfaced, a fleeting yet familiar taste of rock star treatment.

Armed with materials from Are Vaccines Safe, I set up a modest station adjacent to Brandy Vaughan's organization, "Learn the Risk" It was imperative to emphasize that my intentions were altruistic—I gave away cards rather than profiting from them. Like bullets in an army, the cards were dispensed freely to empower those who joined the cause.

Amidst the bustling scene, fellow vendors hawked their wares—t-shirts, books, and sundries—a marketplace of shared advocacy.

Although the room could have accommodated 200 souls, a mere 75 gathered, reminiscent of past events where attendance fell short of expectations, a pang of disappointment tugging at my heartstrings.

The roster of speakers bore unfamiliar names, faces yet to be etched in my memory. In retrospect, they were vital cogs in Del Bigtree's inner circle, figures that now find recognition in the annals of my journey.

A half-hour elapsed, tinged with anticipation, as whispers of Bigtree's imminent arrival circulated. Then, like a thunderclap, the announcement echoed—a mere 15 minutes separated us from his presence.

The colossal black bus maneuvered into view, the herald of change carrying with it Del Bigtree. A roar of applause engulfed the room as attendees surged forward, seeking selfies and handshakes.

My moment neared; I queued up, nerves and excitement twining within me. Thirty minutes later, our eyes met—a culmination of dreams and aspirations. My hand extended, and a handshake ensued, followed by a warm embrace. His stature was not imposing, a revelation that defied my expectations. His teeth bore the marks of time, and a hint of tobacco lingered in the air. Surprisingly, his physique lacked the vigor I envisaged—soft, almost lacking muscle tone.

In that fleeting encounter, I was swept away, the euphoria akin to a girl basking in the presence of the Beatles. Bigtree wielded the potential to reshape the world, and I was determined to join his crusade, to lend my voice to the chorus of change, all in the name of Weston and Emily's memory. I

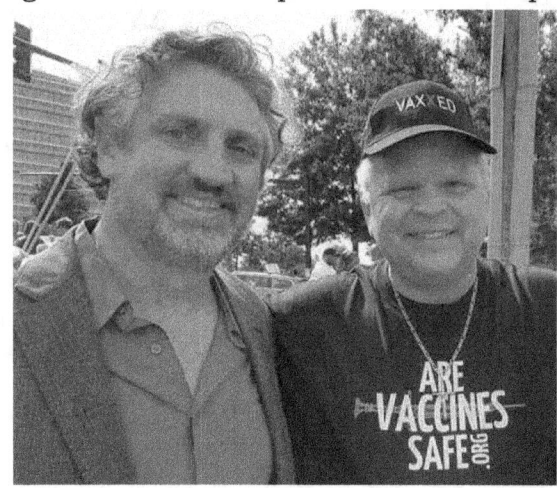

wanted every promise they made to come true, and I was ready and willing to do the grassroots work necessary to ensure it all came to pass.

As our paths converged, I confronted the unexpected—realizing that those who wield transformative power need not fit the mold we envision.

Chapter 5

Family Showmanship

EXCLUSIVE EXPOSE:
DEL BIGTREE'S FAMILY SECRETS

Hold onto your hats as we delve deep into the tantalizing tapestry of Del Bigtree's family history. Prepare for a jaw-dropping ride through a saga that blurs the lines between reality and showmanship, where the truth is a tantalizing enigma waiting to be unraveled. From riveting revelations to shocking twists, this is a story that will leave you craving more.

Step into the spotlight as we peel back the layers of Del's enigmatic background.

A LEGACY OF SHOWMEN

Let's kick off with a bang—Del's family history reads like a script from Hollywood's golden era. A lineage steeped in showmanship and theatrics, where the distinction between the stage and real-life blurs into a mesmerizing dance. Prepare to be mesmerized as we uncover Del's mask in public and the intriguing stories beneath.

Enter stage left, his mother: Norma, born on January 14, 1943, to Norman and Mary Bigtree in Syracuse, NY. Norman Bigtree, a machinist for the Chrysler Corporation until his passing in 1971, was no ordinary man. He was a full-blood Iroquois Indian,

Monetizing Misery

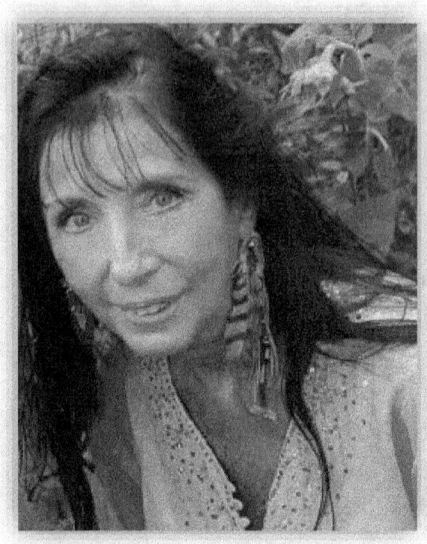

born on the Onondaga Reservation—an ancestry that oozes intrigue. Norma, the eldest of three daughters, would soon find herself treading the boards of the theater world alongside a man named Jack Groverland.

But wait, the plot thickens! Norma's theatrical journey started at age 4 and takes a surreal turn as she stars in Curley McDimple, a Shirley Temple spoof, sharing the limelight with luminaries like Barry Manilow and Bernadette Peters. A star-studded saga that leaves us questioning—did the allure of the spotlight run through Del's veins from the very beginning?

And then came the tumultuous era of "Tent Revival" preaching, a phenomenon that swept the 1960s. Norma and Jack pivoted from thespian glory to the pulpit, trading the theater for the tent in a bid for divine success. A transformation that casts an enigmatic shadow over

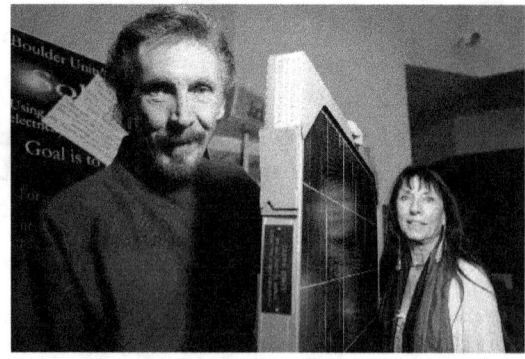

Del's origins and beckons us to untangle the threads of this captivating revival of causes being heralded for fame and fortune.

INTRIGUE BEYOND BLOODLINES

The Bigtree intrigue is far from over. Let's delve into Norman's origins and heritage, a tale that unfolds across continents and defies conventional wisdom. Remember, Norman is Del's grandpa, but to understand the family tree, we will travel back in time.

Norman's heritage echoes the whispers of Native American roots—a captivating claim that evokes the imagery of Iroquoian-speaking tribes. Yet, the narrative acquires a tantalizing twist as sources weave a web of confusion around his lineage. Was Norman truly a full-blooded Iroquois Indian, or did the allure of showmanship extend to the intricacies of his own story?

Norman's ancestral legacy is riddled with questions. Mitchell Bigtree, born in 1876, emerges as a pivotal figure in this saga. A lineage traced back to Philip Bigtree, whose roots intertwine with the heart of Native American heritage, conjuring a legacy that ignites our imaginations.

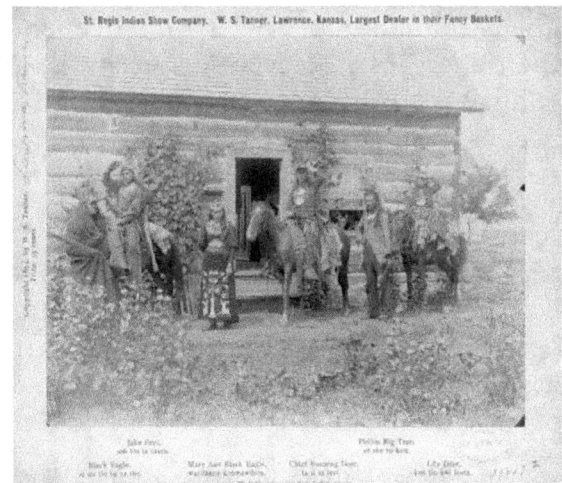

TWO WORDS, ONE MYSTERY

A linguistic dance ensues as Norman's name oscillates between "Bigtree" and "Big Tree," a grammatical enigma that fuels our intrigue. A subtle detail hints at a more significant narrative lurking beneath the surface—record compels us to question the essence of identity and ancestry.

UNRAVELING THE ENIGMA

Norman's tale takes us from the Onondaga Reservation to foreign shores, where echoes of an English marriage cast an enchanting spell. The whispers of Norman's Native American heritage intertwine with the allure of European lineage, creating a tale that defies expectations.

But hold the presses! A grand revelation takes center stage—the lineage of Del's mother, Norma. An ancestry that spans from England to Germany, igniting questions about the mosaic of Norman's ancestral makeup. The enigma deepens as we explore the rich tapestry of Norma's heritage, a narrative that challenges preconceived notions and beckons us to peer beyond the veil of history.

As the curtain falls on this riveting chapter, we recap the tale that has left us spellbound. The tapestry of Del's origins is a complex weave of Native American whispers, theatrical allure, and the intoxicating dance between truth and showmanship. Norma's lineage, a fusion of English and American threads, adds layers of intrigue to this saga of enigmatic proportions.

Prepare for a journey that is far from over. The Big Tree family secrets remain shrouded in mystery, an intricate mosaic waiting to be unraveled. Stay tuned as we venture deeper into the labyrinth of Del's heritage, a narrative that promises twists and turns beyond your wildest imagination. The apple truly doesn't fall far from the Big Tree.

Monetizing Misery

Chapter 6

A Tinseltown Tale of Chiefs and Silver Screens

Buckle up, for the plot takes an electrifying twist! According to my audacious insights, the whispers of Del's lineage lead to none other than the legendary Indian Chief and Hollywood icon—John Big Tree, also known as Isaac Johnny John, who lived from June 2, 1877 – July 6, 1967. Picture this: a silver screen luminary who graced 59 Hollywood films from 1915 to 1950, embodying the very essence of the Indian Chief immortalized on the iconic nickel coin.

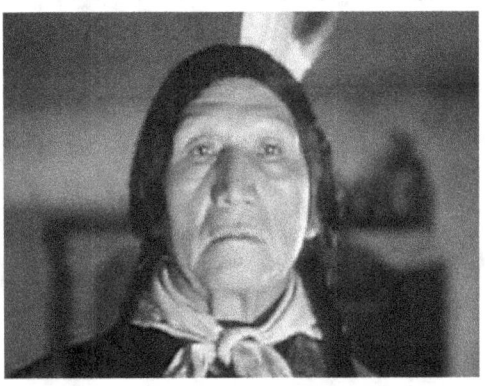

But hold your applause, for confusion casts its shadow over the tale. As we navigate the treacherous waters of online message boards, the Bigtrees and the Big Trees emerge as puzzling protagonists, each vying for their place in the spotlight. My astute observations shed light on the enigma, revealing a tapestry woven with threads of contradiction and intrigue.

A SHOWBIZ PUZZLE: LOST TRUTHS AND AGENDAS

I unraveled a web of contradictions while looking down this path. An obituary of Chief John Big Tree hints at a legacy devoid of progeny—a stark contrast to the whispers of Norma's schoolmate, who remains unnamed and claimed a connection to the illustrious Chief. The essence of truth seems to waver, much like a mirage in showbiz's spotlight.

As the plot thickens, the spelling metamorphoses from Big Tree to Bigtree, introduces a layer of confusion over the narrative. The insidious allure of selling an image emerges as a masterful puppeteer, manipulating the truth in the throes of fame. While Big Tree to Bigtree seems a small stretch, it is two surnames becoming one, and the likelihood of foul play and mistaken identity seems to be amiss.

A TANGLED LEGACY OF LOVE AND LIES

There's more intrigue beneath the surface! Chief John's marital decisions unfold, revealing a tableau of unions and offspring rivaling any Hollywood drama. As if plucked from a script, Chief John's three marriages reveal secrets and surprises that defy expectations.

Chief John's love story unfurls with Phoebe White, a connection that bore fruit in the form of a child named Deforest Johnny John. His tryst with Clara T. Jimerson added another chapter to this riveting tale, birthing Birdie Johnny John.

Yet, there's an even more bewitching twist. Enter Cynthia Johnson Big Tree, an equal suffragist and Indian Model whose union with Chief John birthed no heirs. A final act of love and union that leaves us yearning for answers. Why is he listed as being the father of none when we found two legitimate children from earlier marriages? Are there illegitimate children that might have been given his name without him having been a steady

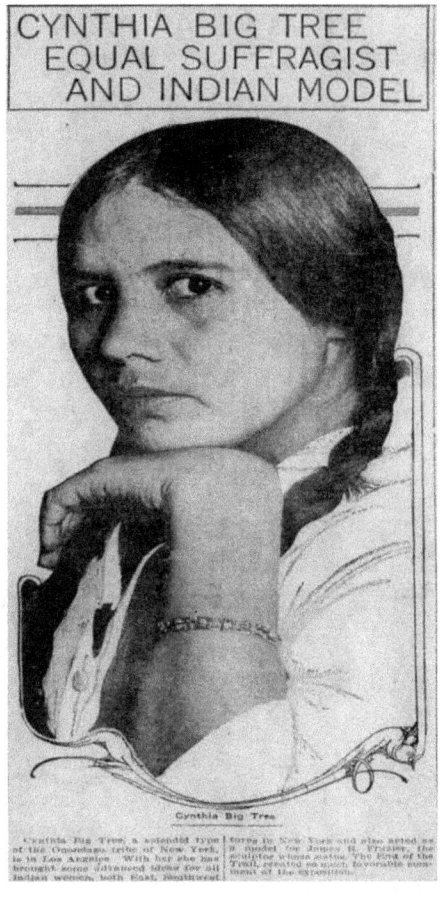

presence in their lives? His marriage record seems to imply that he didn't stay in one set of arms for too long, not even for his children, so is it a safe assumption that the Bigtrees might actually hold relation with Big Tree?

THE CURTAIN CALL: THE MYSTIQUE CRUMBLES

As the plot thickens and the spotlight dims, a tantalizing thread emerges—a potential connection between Chief John and Mitchell Bigtree, Del's forebearer. A tantalizing possibility that sends ripples of speculation through the narrative, leaving us yearning for a grand reveal.

Alas, a chilling reality sets in as the tale reaches its crescendo. Despite my fervent attempts, the enigmatic Miles Mathis remains silent, a conductor who refuses to lead us through this labyrinth of intrigue.

We've come to a crossroads of revelations, shedding light on the intricate tapestry of Norma's ancestry. Norman, her father, emerges not as the full-blooded Iroquois whispered by some sources, but a figure whose lineage weaves a more complex story. The shifting sands of his name, oscillating between "Bigtree" and "Big Tree," cast shadows of confusion, hinting at a potential link to the enigmatic Chief John Big Tree.

In this maze of ancestry, we encounter a grandmother whose roots are firmly planted in British soil, gracing the peerage with her presence. Chief John Big Tree, a figure of both mystique and Hollywood allure, beckons from the depths of history. His connection to the Onondaga Reservation, his birth mirroring that of Mitchell Bigtree, Del's great-grandfather, conjures an uncanny alignment of time and space.

Amidst this sea of information, one thing remains certain: the legend of Norma as the granddaughter of a Mohawk Chief, whose likeness graced the nickel coin, persists through multiple sources. Yet, as we peel back the layers, we uncover the intricate dance of facts and fictions. Mitchell's role as a Mohawk Chief is debunked, replaced by the reality that Chief John Big Tree's likeness adorns the coin in question.

The threads of intrigue are woven intricately, leaving us at a juncture of speculation and uncertainty. The stage is set for Del's potential kinship with Chief John, a hypothesis built on a delicate foundation of shared timelines, geographical echoes, and whispers of ancestral connections. However, the narrative remains woven from strands of coincidence, potential, and the elusiveness of truth. Whether the strands unite in a mosaic of lineage or diverge as mere happenstance, the story remains enshrouded in ancestry's dance.

Chapter 7

Del's Father: Who is the Real Jack Groverland?

FROM ARNEBOLD TO GROVERLAND

The story of Jack Groverland takes an intriguing turn as we delve into the core of his identity. A crucial revelation unfurls: Groverland isn't the name he was born with; he shed his original surname, Arnebold. A key piece of the puzzle emerges with the discovery of his brother's death record, introducing us to his sisters, Katherine and Irene, and hinting at a mother named Sally. The shadowy figure of Sally becomes a lingering enigma, despite the lack of information on Ancestry.com.

FRITZ ARNEBOLD: A GLIMPSE INTO JACK'S FAMILY

Further exploration of Jack's past brings us face-to-face with his father, Frederich "Fritz" Arnebold. Fritz's journey spans from his roots in Germany to his role as a truck driver in the United States under the employment of Charles Miller & Co. His story infuses Jack's lineage with a sense of traversing unfamiliar terrain and shaping a new destiny.

THE CLOUDED ESCAPE: JACK'S BOLD JAILBREAK

In an excerpt from his bio on UnityofBoulder.com, Jack says: "I grew up in the crime infested ghettos of Hoboken and Jersey City where I learned all the wrong ideas about life. I lived with my father, an immigrant truck driver who couldn't begin to imagine the life I'm living now. In those dark days I was a petty thief, gang fighter, gambler and fool. I left all that when I escaped from jail under a hail of bullets and in the process had my first spiritual experience."

Yet, a shroud of uncertainty envelops Jack's narrative, as his daring escape from jail amidst a hail of bullets raises eyebrows and intrigue. The very nature of this escape hints at a life colored by risk and uncertainty, potentially painting him as a fugitive. The motivations behind his name change remain veiled, urging us to uncover the hidden layers beneath the surface. Like father, like son.

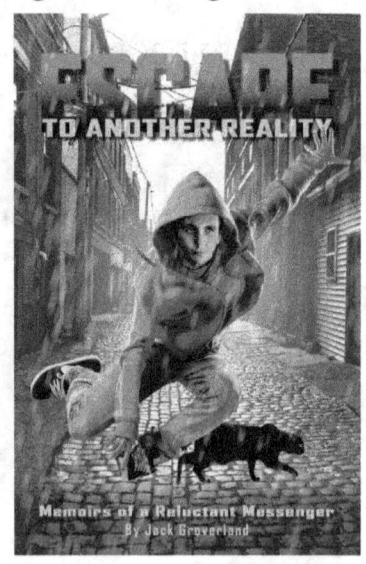

FROM MINISTER TO WORDSMITH

As time unfolds, Jack Groverland wears multiple hats, with each role leaving its mark. From an ordained Unity minister who led the Unity of Boulder community for a remarkable four decades, he seamlessly transitions into a skilled writer whose words resonate far beyond the written page. His literary prowess gives life to books and a screenplay that finds its place in the vibrant realm of Hollywood.

Chapter 8

Del's Wife: Lee Collette Nestor

As our story unfolds, a new chapter brings us to a union that transcends distances and ties two lives together. Del's journey intertwines with Lee Collette Nestor, a meeting that sets the stage for genuine affection and connection. Lee, born on September 23, 1969, in Switzerland, adds an international hue to the narrative.

LEE'S ANCESTRAL LINE

The story of Lee's lineage reveals Peggy Nestor as her mother, but the story runs deeper. Aunts often hold tales of their own, and in Lee's case, Marianne Nestor, known fondly as Dolly, emerges with her own networks. Dolly's connection as the secret wife of fashion luminary Oleg Cassini adds a layer of fascination to the family tale.

PEGGY'S CREATIVE INFLUENCE

Peggy, Lee's mother, the creative visionary behind the Oleg Cassini brand, steps into the limelight. Her role as creative director echoes through the brand's history. Why does this matter? Let's take a look at who Oleg Cassini was.

The glittering world of Oleg Cassini, famed fashion designer, casts a shadow of controversy that goes beyond the runway. In the realm of relationships, his life reads like a gripping tabloid tale.

After a divorce that rocked the headlines, Cassini's romantic journey continued with names that spark curiosity. A chapter intertwined with Gene

Tierney, Hollywood icon, painted a cordial picture even after Gene's 1991 passing. But the allure of Hollywood also led him to the captivating Grace Kelly. An engagement that set tongues wagging hinted at a love story that never reached its publicized crescendo.

Amidst the glamour, a cloud of darkness looms. In an explosive revelation, Susanna Moore bravely alleged that she was subjected to a haunting encounter with Cassini.

The narrative takes an unexpected turn as Cassini's life story intertwines with model Marianne Nestor in a secret marriage. Together, they embarked on a venture that blended fashion and fame. Marianne (pictured to the right with Cassini) took the reins of 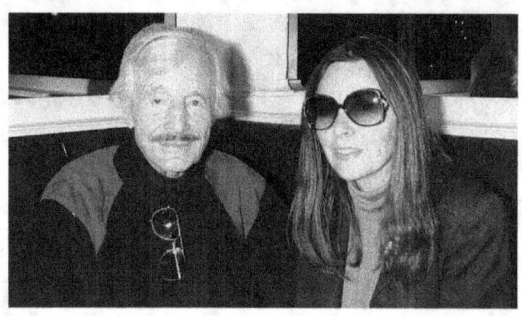 licensing and public relations, igniting a journey that would be remembered for their steadfast defense.

However, their marriage remained cloaked in secrecy until after Cassini's departure from the limelight. What followed was a tumultuous legal showdown that left Marianne and his daughter Tina entangled in a bitter court battle for his estate. The saga captured the public's fascination, with Vanity Fair and Newsday providing updates on the ongoing struggle.

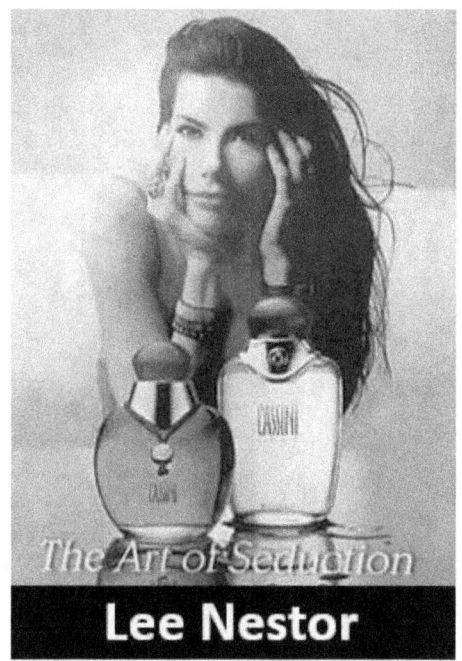

As the pages turned, Cassini's estate took center stage. The year 2019 marked a defining moment as Doyle auctioned off his legacy. The grand finale echoed the complexity that surrounded his life, a chapter that symbolized the culmination of fashion, fame, and fierce legal battles.

Monetizing Misery

Chapter 9

The Kennedy Connection

"Oleg, you are, and will be in fashion history, the designer who created the indelible and stylish image for the First Lady. You should be proud of your achievement, you are the designer who inaugurated her style."

—*Suzy Menkes Fashion Editor; International Herald Tribune, 2003*

OLEG CASSINI

The mention of Oleg Cassini weaves a connection to Jacqueline Kennedy, an icon whose elegance influenced an era. This influence set the stage for a connection between the Nestor family and the Kennedy lineage, establishing a bridge that would eventually bring Del into the fold.

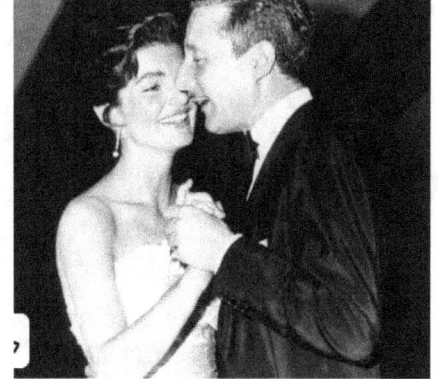

In the corridors of fashion history, Oleg Cassini's name resonates as the virtuoso who draped Jacqueline Kennedy in an aura of timeless elegance. Appointed as her exclusive couturier in 1961, he earned the illustrious title of her "Secretary of Style." This role wasn't just about dresses; it was about defining a legacy.

Cassini's words echoed with prophetic weight when he hailed the dawn of a new American elegance, a sentiment ignited by Mrs. Kennedy's beauty and poise. As her chosen couturier, he held the brush to paint the canvas of the First Lady's iconic look. He embraced French couture techniques and opulent fabrics, weaving them into designs that championed clean lines, crisp forms, and unapologetic luxury.

The "Jackie look" became a global phenomenon, a beacon of sophistication that women worldwide emulated. Cassini's vision wasn't just about clothing; it was about creating an American Queen. Jackie Kennedy, in turn, acknowledged his transformative touch, stating, "Oleg dressed me for the part." Their collaboration birthed an era of fashion that left an indelible mark on history.

Senator Edward Kennedy's words capture the essence of Cassini's impact—his remarkable talent acted as a cornerstone for the New Frontier, setting the stage for iconic changes in fashion. Together, they created style classics that continue to radiate elegance across time.

Cassini's connection with Mrs. Kennedy turned women of all ages into devotees of his art. From 18 to 80, they sought to replicate the allure of geometric dresses and pillbox hats. Meticulously tailored ensembles boasted oversized buttons and boxy jackets, with occasional moments of dramatic décolletage that added a touch of allure.

Among his notable creations, a coat crafted from leopard pelts and a Swiss double satin white gown adorned with a single cocarde stand tall. The latter, worn to the Inaugural Gala Ball in 1961, marked Mrs. Kennedy's official debut as First Lady Elect. Little did they know that this piece would earn its place among the "50 Dresses that Changed the World," an honor bestowed by England's Design Museum—a testament to the enduring impact of Cassini's artistry.

IGOR CASSINI INDICTED

Count Igor Cassini Loiewski emerges as a character entwined with shadows and secrets. Born into the aristocratic legacy of Count Alexander Loiewski and Countess Marguerite Cassini, his story dances between glamour and controversy, leaving a trail of fascination in its wake.

FROM ARISTOCRACY TO STARDOM

Count Igor Cassini's life assumed a multifaceted form, juxtaposing roles that

Igor Cassini Indicted In Lobbying

By TAD SZULC
© New York Times News Service

Washington, Feb. 8. — Igor Cassini, a New York society columnist and international publicity agent, was indicted Friday by a federal grand jury for "willfully and unlawfully" failing to register as an agent for the former Trujillo dictatorship in the Dominican Republic.

Attorney General Robert F. Kennedy said Cassini "assertedly shared in nearly $200,000 in payments from the Dominican Government" resulting from separate contracts in 1959 and 1960 and again in 1961.

Although the Justice Department's announcement of the indictment made no mention of it, documents obtained by The New York Times from the Trujillo archives in Santo Domingo showed that while Cassini was negotiating the 1961 contract he went on a highly confidential mission to the Dominican Republic for President John F. Kennedy.

spanned the worlds of high society and celebrity. He orchestrated his existence as a publicist in the glittering realm of Hollywood's elite, lending his skills to the enigmatic realm of fame. The renowned *Celebrity Register* found its captain in him, while a brief yet impactful stint as the editor of "Status" showcased his literary prowess.

Guided by family bonds, Igor assumed the co-director chair at the House of Cassini, a prestigious fashion company founded by his elder brother, Oleg Cassini. A testament to his charismatic aura, he stepped onto television screens during the 1950s and 1960s, leaving an indelible imprint as a television personality.

FALL FROM GRACE: A FAMILY AFFAIR

The tale took an unexpected twist as the shadows of political intrigue cast their net. Convicted of being a paid agent of Dominican Republic dictator Rafael Trujillo, Igor was ensnared in legal troubles. A conviction for failing to register, as demanded by U.S. law, shattered his world.

The web of connections intricately tied Igor to the Kennedy Administration, a revelation that stirred speculation. The threads of influence woven by his brother, Oleg, known as one of the favorite dress designers of First Lady Jacqueline Kennedy, added a layer of enigma to the narrative.

Amidst the glamour and controversy, Igor's life bore its own tragedies. His union with Charlene Stafford Wrightsman, an oil millionaire's daughter, weaved a story of love and complexity. A marriage marked by turmoil, they became entangled in the whirlwind of Dominican Republic affairs, facing the storm of legal indictments.

In the shadows of Igor's legal battles, Charlene's heartache deepened. A distraught soul, she swallowed thirty sleeping pills, leaving behind a chilling tale. As the 35th Academy Awards flickered on the television screen, her stepdaughter, Marina Cassini, witnessed the tumultuous turn of events. The next day, Charlene's life extinguished, her departure an echoing tragedy.

Chapter 10

Exposing Del Bigtree

Del Bigtree's life traverses the realm of showbiz. From ventures in the risqué world of film to his ascendancy in the VaxXed movement, his career raises questions as to whether any message he is conveying is authentic or sponsored.

FROM STEAMY PRODUCTIONS TO PRODUCERS' GUILD

Del's cinematic journey commences with directorial exploits that stray from the conventional. In 2003, he helmed "Partners," a provocative short film featuring his wife, Lee Nestor. The storyline, entangled in sensuality, exemplifies Hollywood's penchant for pushing boundaries. In 2005, Del donned the dual hats of executive producer and director for "Bitter Sweet," offering a glimpse into his fascination with unconventional narratives.

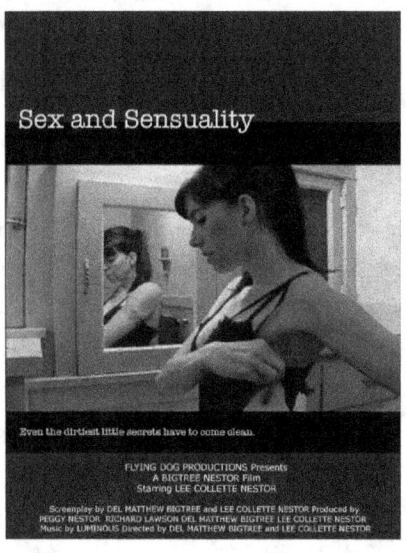

The camera's allure led Del and Lee to co-produce and co-direct "Sex and Sensuality" in 2007, a film brimming with charged undertones. Pegged as a family affair, Lee's mother, Peggy Nestor, joined the production fold. The film's themes of intimacy and secrets added a layer of intrigue, inviting audiences to delve into Del's unique creative vision, including Masonic symbolism. Eyes that can see will.

TELEVISION STINTS AND TANGLED VISION

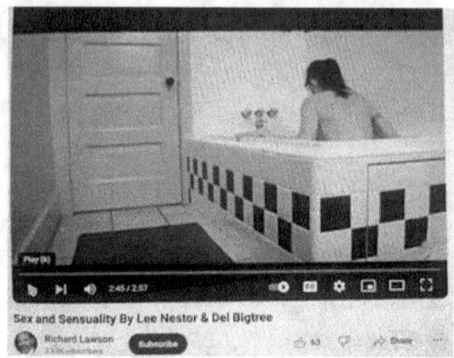

Del's foray into television saw him produce 32 episodes of the widely known show "The Doctors" between 2010 and 2015. The show's pro-pharmaceutical stance didn't deter Del, but his journey was met with a twist when his contract was not renewed in 2015.

Then emerged a significant pivot – Del's involvement in "VaxXed: From Coverup to Catastrophe." His journey intersected with the film's creation when it was over 80% complete, merging his path with the vaccine controversy. A fateful encounter with Andrew Wakefield through mutual connections paved the way for their collaboration, transforming the movie's narrative that so many anti and ex-vaxxers are familiar with.

FROM HOLLYWOOD TO VACCINE CONTROVERSY

Del's influence began to ripple with his additions to the film, incorporating footage from California's Senate Bill 277 rally and interviews with self-proclaimed whistleblower Brandy Vaughan. By March 2016, the final product emerged, but Del's journey was far from over.

Seizing the reins, Del spearheaded the movie's rollout and Q&A sessions, paving the way for a significant shift in his career. A tussle for control ensued, culminating in Andrew's departure and a series of lawsuits. Del's determination to steer the narrative highlighted his commitment to a cause that extended beyond the silver screen, so it seemed.

PURPLE THREADS

Del's path, marked by career metamorphoses, holds undertones of Hollywood's mystique. His penchant for wearing purple, recognized as a Masonic color, adds a layer of intrigue to his story. Purple's symbolism within Masonic circles raises questions about his affiliations and motivations, echoing the enigmatic undertones that surround him. Seemingly, the freedom health movement doesn't delve deeply into Del's associations and past. He gets a mostly free pass as he poses for pictures with fans that get him facial recognition he didn't possess while he was pro-pharma. Good business advice is to find your niche, and it seems he had found his.

Monetizing Misery

Chapter 11

Del Bigtree: A Wolf in Sheep's Clothing

Del Bigtree, a prominent figure in the vaccine safety movement, has built a significant platform advocating for safer vaccines. However, his stance on making vaccines compulsory, if deemed safe, raises severe concerns and contradictions. This chapter delves into how his position conflicts with fundamental personal autonomy and choice principles and why it aligns more closely with pro-vaccine interests than genuine vaccine safety advocacy.

THE SUPREME COURT'S STANCE ON VACCINES

In a landmark decision, the United States Supreme Court labeled vaccines as "unavoidably unsafe." This ruling acknowledges that, despite their benefits, vaccines carry inherent risks that cannot be entirely eliminated. It also supports the notion that individuals should have the right to make informed choices about their health and medical treatments, given the potential for adverse effects.

BIGTREE'S CONTRADICTORY STANCE

Del Bigtree's assertion that vaccines should be made compulsory if they are deemed safe contradicts the Supreme Court's recognition of vaccines as inherently risky. His position undermines the very foundation of the vaccine safety movement, which champions the right to informed consent and personal choice. By advocating for compulsory vaccination, Bigtree supports removing personal autonomy in health decisions. This stance aligns more with pro-vaccine mandates than with advocating for safety and choice.

THE ILLUSION OF SAFETY AND COMPULSION

Bigtree's argument presupposes that vaccines can be entirely safe, which is idealistic and unrealistic. Vaccine manufacturers, driven by profit motives, have historically prioritized financial gain over exhaustive safety measures. The idea that these companies would suddenly produce entirely safe vaccines if they knew how overlooks the complexities of vaccine development and the financial dynamics at play.

PERSONAL AUTONOMY AND CHOICE

Personal autonomy in healthcare is a fundamental right. It encompasses the freedom to make informed decisions about medical treatments based on individual risk assessments and personal beliefs. Compulsory vaccination, even under the guise of improved safety, strips away this autonomy and imposes a one-size-fits-all approach to public health. Bigtree's stance undermines this principle by suggesting that individual choice becomes irrelevant if vaccines are made safe—a position that disregards the nuances and ethical considerations of medical freedom.

A PRO-VACCINE WOLF IN SHEEP'S CLOTHING

Bigtree's platform, while ostensibly advocating for vaccine safety, appears to have deeper implications. His call for compulsory vaccination, contingent on perceived safety, aligns suspiciously well with pro-vaccine mandates. This position serves to placate both vaccine manufacturers and regulatory bodies by promoting the idea that improved safety measures would justify eliminating personal exemptions. It reveals a potential alignment with the entities the vaccine safety movement seeks to hold accountable, positioning Bigtree as a wolf in sheep's clothing.

Del Bigtree's advocacy for compulsory vaccination, based on enhanced safety, conflicts with the core values of personal choice and autonomy. It disregards the inherent risks acknowledged by the Supreme Court and the practical realities of vaccine development. By promoting a stance that ultimately supports vaccine mandates, Bigtree aligns more closely with pro-vaccine interests than with genuine vaccine safety advocacy.

SECTION 2

Divulging the "Game"

Chapter 12

Examining Tactics: Who are the Puppets and Provocateurs in the Web of Psuedo-Resistance?

In psychological warfare and propaganda, Hollywood often serves as a potent tool for crafting and disseminating narratives. It's a realm where illusion blurs with reality, and narratives can shape public opinion. At the heart of this complex web is the enigma of controlled opposition. It is a term and title that gets thrown around often but needs to be dissected to correctly name the players. This book requires that we are all operating from the same definitions for you to draw your own conclusions. Let's dive into controlled opposition and gain more understanding

THE SHADOW PLAY OF DISSENT

Imagine a grand theatrical production where the forces of power choreograph every move, every word, and every dissenting voice. In this carefully scripted drama, controlled opposition takes center stage.

THE PUPPET THEATER

Controlled opposition is like a puppet theater, where the puppeteers are hidden in the shadows, pulling the strings of seemingly independent figures. Often charismatic and persuasive, these figures represent dissent against the established order. They appear to challenge the status quo, but beneath the surface, they are guided by the forces they claim to oppose.

A MIRAGE RESISTANCE

Picture a desert oasis shimmering in the distance, offering hope to weary travelers. This oasis is controlled opposition. It appears to be a source of resistance and alternative perspectives, but as travelers draw closer, they realize it's a mirage. This clever illusion ultimately guides them back into the desert of conformity. Unfortunately, much like a mirage, by the time you reach the seeming oasis, resources and resistance have run out. Unable to fight the proverbial desert of propaganda and misinformation, this is where people will give into agendas they oppose because the will to keep moving has left them.

Sadly, throughout the C-19 narrative, I watched as many people succumbed to taking the jab to keep their jobs, be able to travel, or they simply fell into fear of the 'virus' because of the media frenzy ticking death tolls and horrifying statistics on all screens non-stop.

ORCHESTRATED DISSENT IS THE SAFETY VALVE

Orchestrated dissent serves a dual purpose. It provides an outlet for public dissent, allowing people to express their frustrations and concerns. However, this outlet is carefully channeled, ensuring the dissent stays within the established narrative. It's a safety valve that prevents genuine opposition from gaining momentum.

If you can recollect, many of the "truthers" favorite voices early-on in the Co(n)vid game were decrying the Fauxian agenda while also talking about how terrifying the 'virus' was, citing how the 'virus' was disseminated and destroying the body. This approach did nothing in the way of alleviating fear or garnering movement back to normal society but effectively created an 'us versus them' narrative that pitted 'anti/ex-vaxxers' against the rest of society—those on the fence, uninformed, or pro-vaccine.

WHERE DECEPTION IS AN ART FORM

In this grand theatrical production, deception is an art form. Controlled opposition figures may espouse partial truths to gain credibility. They might even challenge certain aspects of the official narrative. Yet, this is part of the script – a calculated maneuver to maintain the illusion of opposition while never truly undermining the status quo.

It is common for these figures to make impassioned pleas for your safety, drawing you in under their protective wing. This builds a connection, or more clearly, a trauma bind to the controlled opp figure which makes disentangling from their information much more difficult. Why would anyone want to turn away from someone who is risking their public career to bring the truth to the forefront? Except, the sleight of hand is this: their popularity grows and their feigned censorship doesn't keep their message away, it is just enough of dangling the carrot in front of the donkey to make people scream 'foul' from the rooftops and build an enlarging audience for the controlled opposition narrative. If the message were truly a threat, there would be no way to share their information or videos on social media, as many of us found ourselves being deplatformed and silenced throughout the tirade.

Before looking at a deplatforming as a source of trust for anyone, take into account the possibility that even that could be scripted by those at the top. If many followers are encountering an issue, like censorship, it would be counterintuitive if one of the leaders didn't experience the same. The outrage of the followers is a great gauge as to how well the ruse is working. While many common people felt the effects of extreme censorship, the fundraising efforts of controlled opposition would not, and again, many fundraisers of normal people were taken down and funds blocked, so seeing a movement become increasingly lucrative and able to afford bigger and better while requesting more and more donations should be a glaring red flag.

CIRCULAR REPORTING

Circular reporting, also known as echo chamber reporting, occurs when a piece of information is repeated across multiple sources without clearly or accurately attributing its origins. This phenomenon creates a reinforcing loop where the info is perpetuated without direct evidence or clarification of its credibility. Typically, this begins with one news outlet publishing a story, which is then disseminated by others, leading to the source being obscured or presumed to possess greater credibility than it does.

As these reports reference one another, there's a risk of overestimating the reliability of the information, making it challenging to trace back to its initial source or to verify the accuracy of the facts presented. Circular reporting can inadvertently amplify rumors, misinformation, or disinformation, influencing public opinion and decision-making.

THE ELUSIVE PUPPET MASTERS

Like master puppeteers operating from behind the curtains, the true orchestrators of controlled opposition remain hidden. These powerful entities, be they governments, corporations, or secret societies, pull the strings to ensure that the dissenting voices dance to their tune. Since 2020, it has been clearer than ever that the web of puppet masters is much larger than most imagined. This was a 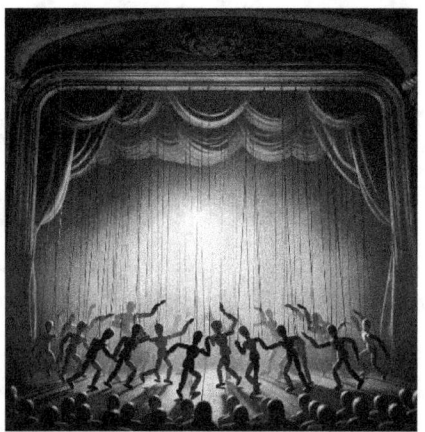 global event that touched (seemingly) every country and caused massive shutdowns across industries. The easy players to peg were governments, pharmaceutical companies, and humongous corporations. There is no need to name any here, all one needs to do is think or look back to who profited during the shutdowns and subsequent years. While small businesses were experiencing crises and shutting down at alarming rates, big corporations saw a soaring bottom line.

THE ILLUSION OF CHOICE

Controlled opposition creates an illusion of choice. It presents two sides of the same coin, giving the impression that the public has alternatives. However, both sides ultimately serve the same interests, ensuring the power structures remain untouched.

The continuing 'Q Agenda' is proof of this with their "Trust the Plan" slogan which has resulted in a tightening noose around the general public's neck. That narrative also divides people within the 'truther' movement. Some full heartedly believe every 'drop,' while others within the same movement are resistant to the agenda. I have seen people from both sides of the fence on the 'Q Agenda' go head-to-head and block each other over their status of belief. And while this book has nothing to do with that separate, if not relevant, narrative, it is a good example of how militant followers of controlled opposition can be.

Any true movement should have mobilization, even (and especially) if the requests are simple but done en masse could affect great change. An example of that is the vaccine information cards I had made up and sent out in the hundreds and thousands so people could hand them out and bring awareness to other parents in the hopes that other families could be diverted from vaccine damage to their beloved children. My goal before, as it is now, has always been to save as many people from harm as I can reach. That's a true grassroots movement

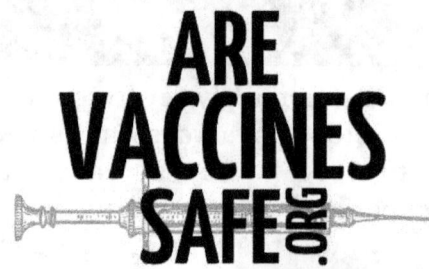

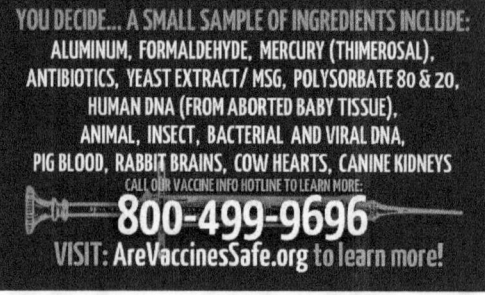

THE STRUGGLE FOR AUTHENTIC DISSENT

In this intricate play, the real struggle lies in discerning genuine dissent from controlled opposition. It requires a keen eye to see beyond the masks, beyond the scripted performances, and to recognize the puppet theater for what it is – a shadow play of dissent, carefully orchestrated to maintain the existing order of things. With all of this in mind, I will share my opinion, though it is my fervent advice that you come to your own conclusions.

Chapter 13

A Quick Recap of How I Got Here

In 2008, I took my first steps into the world of Facebook when it was still in its infancy. My initial purpose was simple: to reconnect with old high school friends. Little did I know that this digital voyage would lead me on an unforeseen expedition, unraveling a story that would define the essence of my existence.

As the years passed, my reasons for using Facebook underwent a profound transformation, aligning with the evolving chapters of my life. It was in 2011 that a new mission began to take shape. I started scouring the platform in search of other parents who, like me, were grappling with the intricate challenges of raising children with autism. This quest was born from deep concern and an insatiable desire to find answers to connect with those who shared my journey.

Yet, a heavy burden of records lay dormant in my closet for several years untouched after the dismissal of Emily and Weston's vaccine court case, until my curiosity got the best of me. These documents held the untold story of my children's medical history, a narrative that would forever alter the course of my life.

Weston's case was filed in 2004, a seven-year odyssey through the legal system that eventually ended in 2011, much like countless others. It wasn't until 2013 that I summoned the strength to face those records. They had remained locked away, suppressed by a gnawing intuition that my suspicions were far from baseless. As I finally pried open those pages, a chilling pattern emerged, revealing a vast cover-up of vaccine injuries.

In 2011, a pivotal moment arrived as a package from the federal government. Weston's medical records were within its confines, a trove of documents previously concealed from my view. The records filled a five-inch three-ring binder. Even then, I hesitated to fully embrace the notion that vaccines could be linked to autism. It seemed inconceivable that the government, an institution I had grown up trusting, could be entangled in such a grave deception that had not only sterilized my father but had now poisoned my children.

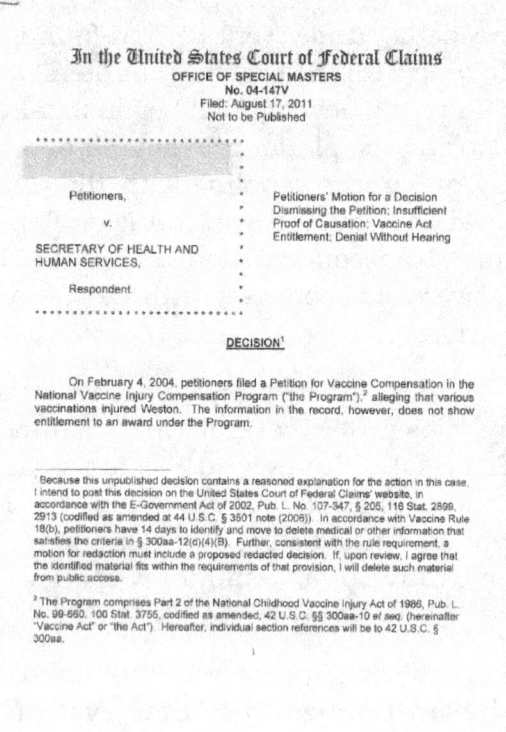

The years rolled on, yet the elusive truth remained beyond my grasp. It wasn't until 2013 or 2014 that the pieces began to fall into place. I was confronted with a reality I had long refused to acknowledge. With a heavy heart and trembling hands, I had locked away those records, unable to entertain the thought that this may have been a deliberate act.

In 2013, life granted me an abundance of time. I returned to Facebook and stumbled upon several parent groups focused on vaccine-injured children. I joined them and was stunned to discover that I was not alone. Thousands of parents, primarily single mothers, searched for answers on Facebook.

By this time, Weston was 15 but looked like a 10-year-old and acted like a 3-year-old. Emily, at 14, behaved like a 6-year-old and was moderately injured. These two beautiful souls, Weston and Emily, would remain eternally young. Caring for them had become an all-consuming task, a responsibility that required the constant support of several caregivers.

Through this tumultuous journey, I met my first close friend, another parent of a vaccine-injured child named Kami Olmstead. Our connection was electrifying, igniting a fire within me to share our stories of children harmed by toxic injections. I began to post relentlessly about Weston and Emily's ordeal, and in doing so, I formed connections with dozens, even hundreds, of friends. The more I shared, the deeper my obsession grew. Facebook became my lifeline.

Kami, a professional businesswoman in 2011 and 2012, had forsaken her career to bring her children's story to the public. With her van packed, she hit the road with her two young vaccine-injured boys, becoming a beacon of hope for those who would listen. She was like a mini-VaxXed bus, and I wouldn't be surprised if Del, of the infamous VaxXed movement, got the idea from her. She was one of the noblest souls I had ever encountered, traversing the Midwest with her own resources, driven by an unwavering love for her children.

Kami's struggle was emblematic of the challenges faced by many parents today. As our children grew older, we grappled with the harsh reality that normalcy was increasingly out of reach. Holding a job became a Herculean task, for our kids had become our full-time responsibility, leaving us with scant time for ourselves.

As the months passed and my knowledge deepened, I became entirely consumed by my mission. I posted incessantly about Weston and Emily's harrowing journey, sharing the documents I had obtained from the vaccine injury court. I scanned and posted them everywhere, driven by a profound sense of purpose. My circle of friends swelled, 95% being mothers; dads were few and far between. Many had succumbed to the unbearable stress, leaving the battle to us, and now, many were in their 30s and 40s that were the bulk of first wave injuries.

I delved into the records alongside my wife, piecing together a narrative that left me dumbfounded. I had no one to confide in about these shocking discoveries back then. It was 2011, and social media, as we know it today, had yet to fully take shape. Facebook was still a lukewarm Myspace, a far cry from the political behemoth it would eventually become.

Undeterred, I continued to join every group I could find, finally stumbling upon Joel Lord and the Vaccine Resistance Movement. It was a group with a solid foundation, a sanctuary for parents of vaccine-injured children.

As I ventured deeper into the world of Facebook parenting groups, a common thread emerged. Our children were born healthy, only to become autistic individuals after vaccinations. As we shared our stories and medical records, the pieces of this intricate puzzle began to fit together. Questions multiplied, and our groups swelled in size. Soon, I was consumed by a relentless pursuit: uncovering the cause of Weston's and Emily's autism.

I painstakingly assembled a timeline of Weston's vaccinations, and what I discovered was nothing short of horrifying. It read like a recipe book of toxic chemicals that had cooked Weston's young brain, leaving me with no doubt. Looking back, realizing something was terribly wrong with what we were doing, and injecting our children with 20 toxic chemicals in their first 90 days of life made me sick. I wondered endlessly: Was this reality, or was I concocting it in my mind? It was a burden that threatened to unravel my sanity.

Driven by an unrelenting passion, I have always sought to change the world to leave an indelible mark on humanity. My background, explored in my other book, had fueled this fervor. In 2013, I began to unravel the truth through these groups. Parents who vaccinated their children had autistic kids, while those who didn't remained unscathed. In 1997 and 1998, information about vaccine side effects was scarce, buried within package inserts, and never disclosed when we signed consent forms. The forms presented minimal side effects, such as a fever or a sore arm. The federal government omitted the severe side effects, deeming them rare. My wife Joyce and I did our best, spacing out vaccines and skipping some, but doubts lingered.

In 2014, I delved deep into research, forging connections with countless parents of vaccine-injured children.

And now, here I stand, armed with a newfound wealth of knowledge and a burning determination. The more I dug into the rabbit hole, the clearer it became: predatory pharmaceutical campaigns, insidious legislation, and puppeteered players were preying upon the unsuspecting masses. It was a game, a sinister game, with stakes higher than most could fathom.

Once seen as a beacon of health and healing, the pharmaceutical industry had revealed its darker side. Behind the polished façade of research and development lay a profit-driven machinery that cared little for the well-being of the people it claimed to serve. The colossal marketing campaigns, designed to lure in healthcare professionals and everyday individuals, were predatory. We were all pawns in a grand scheme, unwitting participants in a dangerous gamble.

Legislation, too, had been manipulated to serve the interests of those with deep pockets and ulterior motives. Laws designed to protect the vulnerable had been perverted, bent to the will of powerful lobbyists and their corporate overlords. It was a system rigged against us, a labyrinth of legal jargon and loopholes that left the innocent in the clutches of the guilty.

And then there were the casted players, individuals carefully chosen to carry out the bidding of a shadowy elite. They appeared on television screens and podiums, their words carefully scripted to deceive and deflect. These players, seemingly champions of public health, were the architects of a grand deception. They were the guardians of a status quo that profited from the suffering of countless innocents.

But I was no longer content to be a pawn in this malevolent game. With every revelation, I felt a surge of purpose, a determination to expose the truth to the world. My journey had led me to this pivotal moment, and I was prepared to reveal the playbook of those who preyed upon the vulnerable.

It was time to shine a light on the darkness, to unmask the predators and their tactics. The world needed to know the insidious game plan carefully concealed from public view. With every word I wrote every connection I forged, I was inching closer to revealing the hidden truths and charting a course toward justice.

I was on a mission for Weston and Emily, for all the children who had suffered, and for the countless families who had been torn apart by the machinations of a heartless industry. I had found my purpose and was determined to share the story of Weston and Emily's journey with the thousands of others who had walked this treacherous path.

This was my calling, my final life project, to unveil the predatory forces that had plagued our society for far too long. I was ready to stand up against the darkness, to speak truth to power, and to lead the charge for a brighter, more just future.

Chapter 14

How the Narrative is Manipulated

The narrative is not free of manipulation. What unfolds for the followers is a strategic unveiling, where the spotlight exposes certain unsavory facets of vaccines and their potential harm. Yet, this is no straightforward illumination—it's a skillfully choreographed performance of controlled opposition. Within this intricate dance, an ulterior motive lurks: the identification of dissenting voices, earmarked for future suppression or discrediting. The aim? To masterfully dictate the flow of information surrounding the conspiracy, ensuring that the complete truth remains elusive, just beyond reach.

At the helm of this operation, a hierarchy takes shape. Those at the apex execute covert maneuvers, seamlessly enacting the coded gestures of Masonic and Luciferian affiliations. Meanwhile, other participants find themselves unwittingly caught in the snare—mere pawns of the Controllers. Together, this orchestrated ensemble unveils segments of the conspiracy, calculated to selectively reveal only fragments of the truth, not the entirety.

Beneath the surface, layers upon layers of deception are laid bare. The puppeteers—front groups bearing the imprints of Freemasonry and Illuminati influence—unleash attacks on the very conspiracy they themselves have cultivated. However, there's a predetermined threshold to their revelations. Only specific tiers of the conspiracy are allowed to see the light, leaving much concealed. It's a careful balancing act, a strategic interplay of exposure and concealment, designed to grant the illusion of "credibility" to these groups while they strive to manipulate the overarching narrative.

Should a group emerge, armed with the potential to unveil the conspiracy in its entirety, a response is triggered—a full-scale assault from external forces. Yet, the battleground extends beyond the surface. Wolves, camouflaged as sheep, are dispatched to infiltrate and dismantle from within. A stark caution emerges from this shadowy realm—a warning to those who venture into the realm of absolute exposure, for the same forces that orchestrate controlled opposition are poised to strike. These insidious forces may have already insinuated their influence, lurking in unsuspecting corners, ready to strike at a moment's notice.

In this realm of manipulation, the narrative sways like a pendulum, drawing the unsuspecting into its sway. It's a calculated performance, a delicate web woven with cunning precision. To navigate this intricate dance, one must pierce the veil, unravel the layers of deception, and emerge with a steadfast determination to seek the truth beyond the façade. As the narrative unfolds, one must remain vigilant, for the shadows hold secrets that threaten to obscure the path to enlightenment.

Chapter 15

Unraveling the Financial Schemes of the Health Freedom Movement

In the dismal depths of online censorship, a troubling pattern emerges—a pattern of selective silencing and opportunistic exploitation. While advocates of alternative health therapies decry censorship as a means to silence their message, a deeper examination reveals a sinister truth: a calculated campaign to manipulate the narrative and capitalize on the unwavering loyalty of the followers of Health Freedom Movement "leaders."

The censorship these "leaders" encounter is a smokescreen, masking their intentions and motivations. Yet, as we peel back the layers of deception, we uncover a web of financial schemes and opportunistic profiteering.

Questions stack up as we scrutinize the lavish fundraising efforts of figures like Del Bigtree and his cohorts. Why do they require exorbitant sums of money when the costs of maintaining their online presence are minimal? Why is there a need for constant appeals for donations despite their purported mission of spreading information freely?

The lack of transparency surrounding these financial endeavors raises red flags, yet their followers remain steadfast in their support, seemingly oblivious to the manipulation at play. Monthly donors, caught in the illusion of philanthropy, unwittingly contribute to the enrichment of a select few while the actual beneficiaries of their generosity remain shrouded in secrecy. Some major donors are part of a gigantic money laundering scheme as a front for non-profits and charities that are only started to move money, whether the people at the top care about the cause or not—usually it's an opportunity to exploit a hot topic.

In the end, it is the disenfranchised and the vulnerable who bear the brunt of this exploitation. As the rich grow richer and the poor grow poorer, the illusion of censorship serves as a convenient distraction, diverting attention from the actual beneficiaries of this insidious enterprise.

Chapter 16

Grifters - The Art of Deception

Grifters, a term derived from "grifter" or "grifting," are individuals who engage in various forms of deception, manipulation, and fraud to acquire money, assets, or influence from unsuspecting victims. Grifting is scamming or conning someone out of money or valuable assets through deception or fraud. It typically involves gaining an individual's trust and exploiting it for personal gain. Grifting can take many forms, from small-scale schemes to elaborate and sophisticated scams, and can be perpetrated in person and online.

A grifter is typically characterized by their ability to charm, manipulate, and exploit the trust or vulnerability of others for personal gain. Their tactics range from simple confidence tricks to complex schemes, and they often operate on the fringes of legality.

COMMON TYPES OF GRIFTERS
- Con Artists: Con artists specialize in deception and often use elaborate stories or scams to manipulate victims into giving them money or valuables.
- Cult Leaders: Some cult leaders employ grifting techniques to build devoted followings and extract money, labor, or loyalty from their followers.
- Ponzi Schemers: Grifters who operate Ponzi schemes promise high returns on investments but use funds from new investors to pay

previous investors, creating a financial house of cards.
- ➤ Televangelists: Some televangelists have been accused of exploiting people's faith for financial gain, soliciting donations for purported religious purposes but using the money for personal wealth.

MOTIVATIONS OF GRIFTERS

Grifters are driven by various motivations, including financial gain, power, and the desire for attention or adoration. Understanding these motivations can shed light on the tactics they employ:

- ➤ Financial Gain: Many grifters are primarily motivated by the prospect of accumulating wealth through deception. They prey on the financial vulnerabilities of their victims.
- ➤ Power and Control: Some grifters are motivated by a desire for power and control over others. They manipulate their victims emotionally, psychologically, or spiritually to establish dominance.
- ➤ Validation and Adoration: Grifters often crave validation and adoration. They may be motivated by the admiration or loyalty they receive from their victims, which bolsters their self-esteem.
- ➤ Psychological Satisfaction: Deceiving others can be psychologically satisfying for some grifters. They derive a sense of achievement from their ability to outwit others.

THE IMPACT OF GRIFTERS

The impact of grifters can be far-reaching and devastating, affecting individuals, communities, and even society as a whole:

- Financial Loss: Victims of grifters may suffer significant financial losses, sometimes leading to financial ruin, bankruptcy, or the loss of their life savings.
- Emotional and Psychological Harm: The emotional toll on victims can be profound, including feelings of betrayal, shame, and mistrust. Some victims may also experience long-lasting psychological trauma.
- Undermining Trust: Grifters erode trust within society, making it more difficult for people to trust others, especially in financial or charitable contexts.
- Legal and Social Consequences: Grifters who operate outside the bounds of the law may face legal repercussions, while their actions can lead to heightened skepticism of similar endeavors.

DETECTING AND PREVENTING GRIFTERS

Preventing falling victim to grifters requires vigilance and critical thinking. Key strategies include:

- Skepticism: Maintain a healthy level of skepticism, especially when approached by individuals or organizations promising extraordinary returns or benefits.
- Research: Conduct due diligence and research before engaging with any financial or charitable opportunity. Verify the credibility and authenticity of individuals or entities.
- Legal Protections: Familiarize yourself with laws and regulations that pertain to investments, charitable donations, and consumer protection to better safeguard your interests.

> Education: Educate yourself and others about common grifting tactics and red flags. Awareness is a powerful tool in preventing victimization.

Grifters are skilled manipulators who use deception and charm to exploit the trust and vulnerability of their victims. Understanding their motivations, tactics, and impact is essential for safeguarding oneself and society. While grifters may persist, vigilance, skepticism, and education are vital in preventing their deceitful practices from succeeding.

NOTICING THE BIGTREE GRIFT

I recall vividly the emergence of Bigtree's ventures into grifting. Everywhere you turned, he was soliciting funds for his charities and nonprofits. What struck me as particularly odd was the apparent lack of reciprocity towards the very individuals they purported to assist – those who were already burdened with injured children and shattered lives. It simply didn't sit well with me.

Amid it all, I found myself digging into my pockets, contributing to aid anyone I could. Curiously, I even entertained the idea of joining Bigtree's organization, hoping to facilitate the redistribution of the millions they amassed in donations to those in need. The hypocrisy of it all was staggering, symbolic of the worst facets of humanity.

But now, as I reflect on my journey, I find myself an old man running on fumes. I gave it my all, every ounce of my being. I take matters like these so seriously and care more than most. Empathy has been my lifelong companion, guiding me with a simple mantra: God first, others second, self last.

Chapter 17

Familial Grifting – Passing Down Deception

Familial grifting can sometimes involve the passing down of deceptive tactics and manipulation from one generation to the next. In some cases, grifters may teach their offspring the art of deception and encourage them to enter different arenas or professions that continue the family tradition of exploitation. This chapter explores how familial grifters may groom their children to follow in their deceptive footsteps and exploit various arenas for personal gain.

PASSING DOWN THE ART OF THE GRIFT

Some familial grifters choose to groom their children or heirs to continue their legacy of deception, manipulation, and exploitation. This grooming process can take various forms:

- ➢ Mentorship: Grifter parents may mentor their children, teaching them the tactics and strategies of deception. This can include lessons on manipulating, charming, or swindling others.
- ➢ Ideological Indoctrination: In cases where familial grifting is intertwined with specific ideologies or beliefs, parents may indoctrinate their children into these ideologies, encouraging them to use their inherited beliefs for deception.
- ➢ Training in Deceptive Practices: Parents may directly teach their children the practical

aspects of grifting, including confidence tricks, fraud, or manipulation techniques.
- ➢ Entrance into Deceptive Professions: Familial grifters may encourage their offspring to enter fields where deception and manipulation are prevalent, such as televangelism or the "medical freedom" movement.

EXAMPLES OF FAMILIAL GRIFTING CONTINUITY
- ➢ MLM Marketing/Pyramid Schemes: Family and friend groups make sure that they are the top of the pyramid and that they can change who is at the pinnacle as needed.
- ➢ Televangelism: A televangelist father might encourage his children to follow in his footsteps and continue his ministry. They may be taught how to solicit donations from followers under the guise of religious contributions. Or, a televangelist father might encourage a child to join the:
- ➢ Medical Freedom Movement: A parent involved in the "medical freedom" movement might groom their children to become prominent figures within the movement, using their influence to promote alternative medical practices or sell unproven remedies.

MOTIVATIONS BEHIND PASSING DOWN GRIFTING
The motivations behind passing down the art of the grift to the next generation can vary:
- ➢ Continuation of Wealth: Grifter parents may want to ensure that their family continues to enjoy the financial benefits of deception.
- ➢ Legacy: Some grifters view their deceptive practices as a family tradition or legacy they want their children to uphold.

- Control: Encouraging children to participate in deception can grant parents control over their offspring, as they may rely on their parents for financial or professional success.
- Shared Beliefs: In cases where grifting is tied to specific beliefs or ideologies, parents may see grooming their children as a way to perpetuate those beliefs.

CONSEQUENCES OF PASSING DOWN DECEPTION

Passing down the art of the grift to the next generation can have wide-ranging consequences:

- Family Dysfunction: It can lead to family dysfunction, estrangement, and damaged relationships, as the offspring may resent or disapprove of their parents' actions.
- Continuation of Deception: It perpetuates deception and manipulation, causing harm to others and society at large.
- Legal Consequences: The parent and the child could face legal repercussions if their deceptive practices are exposed.
- Perpetuation of Harmful Beliefs: If deception is tied to harmful or dangerous beliefs, the passing down of these beliefs can lead to real-world harm, mainly when propagated through the next generation.

MAKING CONNECTIONS

Controlled opposition is a concept that often overlaps with grifting but involves a different level of organization and intent. While grifters engage in deceptive practices for personal gain, controlled opposition implies a more calculated approach, where an organization, entity, or government covertly controls or influences an opposition group or movement to serve its objectives. This concept is often associated with political or social contexts, but also happens within friend and family groups, and can be used strategically to manipulate public opinion and maintain control. In the next section, we'll explore controlled opposition in greater detail.

Chapter 18

MLM and Supplement Game— Making Millionaires: The Exploitative Structure of Multi-Level Marketing

In recent years, the term "MLM" or Multi-Level Marketing has garnered both fascination and controversy. Often glorified as a pathway to financial freedom, it's imperative to delve beyond the surface glamour and examine the intricate mechanisms through which MLMs operate. This chapter seeks to dissect the exploitative structure inherent in the MLM and supplement game.

UNDERSTANDING MULTI-LEVEL MARKETING

At its core, multi-level marketing is a hierarchical business model that heavily relies on a network of distributors to sell overpriced products or services. These distributors earn commissions from both their direct sales and also from the sales of those they recruit into the network, forming a hierarchical structure akin to a pyramid. While MLMs often present themselves as opportunities for financial prosperity and personal growth, reality paints a different picture. Thousands of other top-level organizers and founders, high on the wings of the Health Freedom Movement, find a never-ending fertile ground of constant recruits from vulnerable souls looking for love, friendship, and of course, money to deal with the dynamics of vaccine damage that led them to MLM leaders exploiting the Health Freedom Movement.

THE PYRAMID SCHEME RENAMED

One of the defining characteristics of Multi-Level Marketing (MLM) companies is their resemblance to pyramid schemes. The primary focus is often not on the sale of products but on recruitment. Those at the top of the pyramid reap the lion's share of profits, while those at the bottom struggle to make ends meet. Notable individuals in the Health Freedom Movement exemplify those who have ascended to the upper echelons of these pyramids, leveraging their positions to amass wealth at the expense of countless others.

EXPLOITING THE VULNERABLE

The ascent of figures like a "prominent" doctor who peddles supplements with his name on them and his wife who has a sketchy past to MLM millionairedom is not without controversy. The wife, aforementioned, has a checkered past, and transitioned from an ex-prostitute to an MLM mogul, which underscores the predatory nature of such schemes. Similarly, the supplement doctor's empire, built on pseudoscience and misinformation, highlights the ethical quandaries inherent in MLM practices. By preying upon the vulnerabilities of their clientele, these individuals perpetuate a cycle of exploitation under the guise of health and wellness.

VULTURES OF THE HEALTH FREEDOM MOVEMENT

In conclusion, these MLM leaders' practices resemble those of vultures, exploiting society's most vulnerable for their own gain. Their success stories are a stark reminder of the dangers and ethical issues surrounding MLM schemes.

Perhaps the most insidious is MLM proponents' co-optation of legitimate movements, such as the Health Freedom Movement. By positioning themselves as champions of individual rights and wellness advocacy, they manipulate unsuspecting parents into purchasing overpriced products under the guise of empowerment. In doing so, they perpetuate harmful pseudoscience (the virus lies and outrageous claims that their products alone will fix your parasites/heavy metals issues/detoxing/etc.) and erode trust within communities seeking genuine solutions to health concerns.

MLM millionaires, that will remain unnamed but are very active and public online, represent the epitome of exploitation within the multi-level marketing industry. By capitalizing on vulnerable individuals and leveraging deceptive tactics, they perpetuate a cycle of inequality and misinformation. As awareness grows surrounding the true nature of MLMs, it becomes increasingly crucial to scrutinize their practices and hold accountable those who profit at the expense of others.

Chapter 19

The Zeolite Debate: Natural Benefits vs. Synthetic Schemes

UNDERSTANDING ZEOLITES

Zeolites are naturally occurring minerals formed from volcanic ash and seawater over millions of years. These microporous, aluminosilicate minerals have a unique crystalline structure that makes them highly effective at trapping and removing toxins from the body. Zeolites are known for their ability to:

1. Detoxify the Body: Their cage-like structure allows them to capture and bind toxins, heavy metals, and other harmful substances, which are then safely excreted from the body.

2. Improve Gut Health: By removing toxins, zeolites can promote a healthier gut environment, potentially alleviating issues such as leaky gut syndrome.

3. Support Immune Function: Detoxification can improve immune function by reducing the body's burden of harmful substances.

4. Balance pH Levels: Zeolites can help balance pH levels, which is essential for maintaining across-the-board health.

It is important to note that while some studies have shown promising results, more clinical trials are needed to understand the health benefits and safety of ingesting zeolites fully. As with all supplements, it is advisable to consult with a healthcare professional before starting zeolite supplementation.

THE RISE OF SYNTHETIC ZEOLITES AND TRS

With the growing popularity of natural zeolites, the market has seen the emergence of synthetic zeolite products. Synthetic zeolites are engineered in laboratories to mimic the structure and properties of natural zeolites. However, there are significant differences between natural and synthetic zeolites:

1. Manufacturing Process: Synthetic zeolites are produced through chemical processes that can introduce impurities or alter their effectiveness compared to naturally occurring zeolites.

2. Efficacy: Zeolites' natural formation process over millions of years results in a highly stable and effective structure, which can be challenging to replicate accurately in a laboratory setting.

3. Safety: Concerns have been raised about the potential for synthetic zeolites to contain contaminants or have different properties that might pose health risks.

Synthetic zeolites are marketed as powerful detoxification supplements, claiming to offer numerous health benefits. However, these products often come at a high cost. For example, a 1-ounce bottle of synthetic liquid zeolites like TRS can sell for upwards of $90 for a 30-day supply. In contrast, you can purchase a six-month supply of non-synthetic, natural zeolites for a fraction of that cost, about $10 a month. This significant price difference highlights the profit margins involved in synthetic zeolite products.

TRS: A MULTI-LEVEL MARKETING SCHEME

TRS (Advanced TRS) operates as a multi-level marketing (MLM) scheme, which raises several red flags:

1. MLM Structure: TRS is sold through an MLM business model, where individuals buy the product and are encouraged to recruit others to sell it. This structure often prioritizes recruitment over product quality and customer satisfaction.

2. High Costs: Products sold through MLM schemes, including TRS, are typically much more expensive than comparable products from traditional retail channels. This is due to the need to support multiple commission levels within the MLM structure.

3. Questionable Claims: MLM products often exaggerate health claims to entice buyers and recruits. In the case of TRS, claims about its detoxification capabilities and overall health benefits are not always supported by rigorous scientific evidence.

THE USUAL SUSPECTS

Interestingly, many of the same individuals and influencers who promote other controversial health products and MLM schemes are also at the forefront of pushing TRS. These players often have a track record of involvement in various health-related MLM schemes, leveraging their influence and followers to drive sales and recruitment.

- A few obvious names (again, those in the movement will know their names) have become millionaires from their involvement in TRS and other MLM schemes. They operate discreetly to avoid drawing attention to their activities.

- An initial partner in the TRS endeavor, the one guy later was involved with another controversial MLM product called Black Oxygen Organics, which the government eventually shut down. After that failure, he made his own line of products.

BLACK OXYGEN ORGANICS:
A CASE STUDY IN MLM FAILURE

Black Oxygen Organics (BOO) was marketed as a revolutionary health supplement with purported detoxification benefits. People were drinking and bathing in dirt and posting it on social media. The primary reason for Black Oxygen Organics' downfall was the discovery that their products contained dangerous levels of heavy metals, including lead and arsenic. The FDA issued a warning advising consumers not to use BOO's Fulvic Care powder and tablets due to these health risks. There were reports of consumers experiencing adverse health effects, such as persistent headaches, which were linked to the high levels of these toxic substances.

Additionally, the company faced significant legal challenges, including a federal lawsuit and claims of unpaid commissions by its distributors. The negative publicity and regulatory scrutiny ultimately forced Black Oxygen Organics to shut down its operations in late 2021. It is obvious that at least THREE MLMs currently use that bog "fulvic and humic."

BOO operated under a classic MLM structure, promising potential monthly earnings of up to

$144,000. However, the product had no proven benefits, and the scheme was eventually exposed as a scam, leading to its shutdown. The other companies who repackaged the old BOO product remain under the radar only because they have more than one product, so they aren't bringing any scrutiny to their added offering.

While natural zeolites offer promising health benefits, the rise of synthetic zeolites like TRS and their association with MLM schemes should be approached with caution. The MLM model prioritizes recruitment and profit over product efficacy and consumer well-being, often leading to inflated prices and questionable health claims. Consumers should be wary of products promoted through MLM structures and seek information from reliable and independent sources to make informed decisions about their health.

Chapter 20

Controlled Opposition vs. Orchestrated Dissent and Psuedo-Resistance: Manipulating Dissent for Strategic Gains

Controlled opposition is a covert strategy that involves influencing or managing opposition groups, movements, or individuals in a way that serves the interests of a controlling entity. For my purposes, I will call this "orchestrated dissent" and "pseudo-resistance" for the rest of the book, since we don't know who the controllers are, we can only guess. This chapter explores the concept of orchestrated dissent, its historical applications, and a specific example within the context of the "medical freedom" movement.

Controlled opposition is a strategy employed by governments, institutions, or organizations to manipulate dissent and control narratives while maintaining the appearance of a legitimate opposition. Key characteristics include:

- ➤ Covert Control: The controlling entity, often with hidden motives, subtly guides or influences the actions, messaging, and objectives of the opposition group.
- ➤ Maintaining Appearances: The controlled opposition is designed to appear genuine and grassroots, making it difficult for the public to discern the manipulation.
- ➤ Strategic Goals: The controlling entity uses this strategy to achieve specific objectives, such as

neutralizing dissent, diverting public attention, or furthering its agenda.
- ➤ Sowing Division: Controlled opposition may create internal divisions within legitimate opposition movements, weakening their impact.

PSEUDO-RESISTANCE IN THE "MEDICAL FREEDOM" MOVEMENT

Within the realm of healthcare and medical policy, the "medical freedom" movement has been a contentious area where controlled opposition has been alleged. This movement advocates for personal choice in healthcare decisions, often opposing mandatory vaccinations, mask mandates, and other public health measures. A historical example of controlled opposition within this movement involves the perceived influence of particular interest groups and political actors. While we won't specifically name anyone, the inferences are straightforward.

- ➤ Vaccine Skepticism: The "medical freedom" movement has gained momentum with increasing vaccine hesitancy and skepticism about vaccination mandates. While I am a vaccine abolitionist, the "medical freedom" movement has often been found speaking of "safer" vaccines, spacing the scheduled vaccines out more, and tailoring a different schedule. The movement also encourages genetic testing for MTHFR Gene Mutation and others before vaccinating instead of taking the abolitionist approach. There is no way to know, even taking these factors into consideration, which children or people will experience adverse effects. While vaccine skepticism is a start, it is cowardly not to go the entire way and say "no more" unless there is a hidden motive.

➢ Political and Financial Interests: Critics have alleged that political figures and organizations, influenced by political and financial interests, have covertly supported and directed elements of the "medical freedom" movement. This seems evident in the promise to overturn the 1986 Indemnity Act that allowed vaccine manufacturers to incur no financial losses for faulty products while passing the financial burden of their products onto unsuspecting taxpayers. Not only that, the movement has been used as a platform for political hopefuls. The fanbase built within the "medical freedom" movement is now being used to say, "I met him, and he's a great guy," "We're friends, and he cared about my story when I shared it," when it was a photo opportunity to this end--to build political credibility with the average Joe and Jane, akin to kissing babies on a campaign trail.

➢ Manufacturing Doubt: The goal of controlled opposition within the "medical freedom" movement is to manufacture doubt about established scientific consensus regarding vaccines and public health measures. This doubt can lead to reduced public trust in healthcare institutions and policies, which again can be a good thing. The problem is in replacing one problem with one that makes them money and still causes the same harm that the original did. Here, I encourage you to find out who has a financial interest, stake, and something to lose if an alternative choice is kept private.

> Policy Impact: By influencing the movement, controlling entities may shape public policy decisions, such as legislation. Here, controlled opposition is ensuring that old policies stay firmly in place. That is where the problem lies. The 1986 Indemnity Act should be overturned. It was the sole reason I jumped on board the VaxXed Bus movement, thinking the tide was turning in favor of the injured. Untold millions have been raised amidst many legislation promises, yet nothing gets done.

THE IMPACT OF ORCHESTRATED DISSENT

Orchestrated dissent can have several consequences:

> Diminished Legitimacy: Genuine opposition movements may lose credibility as their message becomes associated with manipulated elements. Like the "Trust the Plan" movement, followers are encouraged to sit back and do nothing but financially back the movement so the "experts" can do what they do, which is nothing. The illusion, though, is that all the promises they make on tours will be worked on and attained.

> Eroded Public Trust: Controlled opposition can erode public trust in institutions, especially when it sows doubt and subverts the initial cause of the followers. Vaccine hesitancy and spacing out a lessened vaccine schedule are not the intent of an anti-vax crowd. Easily manipulated, some followers drop their original

flag and start becrying the new epitaph of the movement.

- ➤ Division: Internal divisions and infighting within movements can weaken their overall impact and effectiveness. The "VaxXed" Bus tour seemed to be a uniting factor, and yet so many that signed their names to the bus quietly agreed that something was not quite right. Heaven forbid you speak against one of the visible movement leaders. Their followers will discredit your concerns and fast.

DETECTING AND COUNTERING PSUEDO-RESISTANCE

Detecting and countering pseudo-resistance requires vigilance and critical thinking:

- ➤ Independent Research: Rely on credible sources and conduct independent research to verify information and claims within any movement or group. If their movement doesn't match their claims, ask why. At least withhold donating until you gain clarity on this.

- ➤ Question Motivations: Examine the motivations and potential hidden interests of prominent figures and organizations within the movement. Are any of them running for political office in the past, now, or have plans to run? What was their track record before joining the movement? If it was on a vastly different scale, why?

- ➤ Transparency and Accountability: Promote transparency and accountability within opposition movements to ensure they remain true to their stated goals and principles. But beware, people in this movement call for transparency and accountability while never giving it. This is a bait-and-switch tactic because, in the minds of many people, if they are asking for transparency and accountability, then they must be transparent and accountable. That illusion is a calculated fallacy.

➢ Dialogue and Engagement: Engage in open dialogue and constructive discussions to foster transparency and cohesion within movements. The scripted questions and answers are not the end all be all--it's time for new questions that would have been harder to rehearse. When challenged, controlled opposition will project that label back on the person questioning their legitimacy. They will also play it off with a playful admission.

Controlled opposition is a complex strategy used to manipulate dissent and control narratives. Understanding this concept is crucial for recognizing potential manipulation within movements and maintaining transparency and accountability to address legitimate concerns. By remaining vigilant and promoting open dialogue, individuals and organizations can help safeguard the integrity of opposition movements and protect their ability to advocate for genuine social change.

THE OVERLAP

In examining the worlds of grifters and controlled opposition, it becomes evident that deception, manipulation, and the exploitation of trust are threads woven through the fabric of human behavior and society. Grifters often operate individually and seek personal gain through artful deceit. A handful of grifters that have linked up in purpose and cause will work together while managing different entities, be they businesses but usually non-profits (to evade those taxes). Most people who partner up for a cause and spend considerable time together would also form a business entity as partners. Controlled opposition represents a calculated and organized approach to influence narratives and control dissent for larger strategic objectives. This could be how a group of individuals came to work together.

While these two phenomena may appear distinct, they share common elements. They both challenge the fundamental principles of transparency, honesty, and trust within human interactions. Grifters undermine the bonds of trust among individuals and can leave a trail of broken lives and shattered confidence in their wake. Controlled opposition, on a larger scale, manipulates narratives, blurring the lines between authenticity and deceit, often leading to confusion and division within society.

In recognizing these shared elements, it is essential to remain vigilant, promote critical thinking, and foster open dialogue. By doing so, we can collectively safeguard against the harmful consequences of grifters and controlled opposition. This is my attempt to shield people and open minds and eyes to what is happening before us.

Chapter 21

Charities and Fraudulent Promises - The Illusion of Change

Charities and nonprofit organizations play a crucial role in addressing societal issues and supporting those in need. They often work tirelessly to raise funds, generate awareness, and mobilize resources for their respective causes. However, beneath the noble exterior of charitable endeavors lies a complex and sometimes disheartening truth. This chapter delves into the issues of fraudulent promises and financial mismanagement that can undermine the efficacy of philanthropic efforts.

ILLUSION OF CHANGE

We've seen it repeatedly - documentaries and movements aimed at educating the public and sparking action on critical issues. The promise of change hangs in the air, but often, the only tangible outcome is the enrichment of a few individuals. Charities, founded with the intent of addressing pressing concerns, sometimes become mired in controversy over financial mismanagement and ineffective action. Let's explore this disconcerting pattern:

> ➢ False Promises: Activist movements and documentaries, while stirring our emotions and raising awareness, frequently lead to an assumption that significant change is on the horizon. Unfortunately, these expectations are not always met.

- Financial Gain for Few: Despite the high ideals of these movements, the primary beneficiaries often turn out to be the individuals leading or associated with the charitable organizations established under their banner. They amass considerable wealth while the issues they purportedly address continue unabated.

MOVEMENTS IN THE SPOTLIGHT:
- VaxXed: The controversial documentary "VaxXed," which questioned vaccine safety, failed to halt vaccination or change vaccine formulations. Yet, the associated charities received significant contributions.
- Human Trafficking Documentaries: Documentaries addressing human trafficking may raise public awareness, but the issue persists, while charities involved receive substantial funding.
- BLM and Racial Injustice: Despite the widespread support for the Black Lives Matter movement, racial injustices continue, and charities affiliated with the cause raise substantial sums.
- Animal Welfare, Disaster Relief, Environmental Conservation, and Medical Research: Numerous charities and foundations have been established to combat these issues. However, the problems persist, and the promises of resolution often fall short.

THE CHARITABLE ILLUSION

Charitable organizations exist to make a positive impact on the world, but disillusionment often arises when their practices deviate from their noble missions:

- Questionable Allocation of Funds: Some charities allocate significant portions of their donations to administrative costs and salaries rather than directly aiding the causes they champion.

- Ineffective Programs: Despite their lofty goals, charitable organizations may have ineffective or inefficient programs that fail to bring about the intended change.

- Lack of Accountability: In some cases, the transparency and accountability of these charities come under scrutiny, as it becomes unclear where and how donations are spent.

- Conflict of Interest: The personal interests of those leading these organizations can sometimes overshadow the mission, leading to financial gain at the expense of genuine progress.

The issues surrounding fraudulent promises and the financial mismanagement of charitable organizations underscore the need for transparency, accountability, and rigorous scrutiny within philanthropy. While many charities genuinely strive to effect change, the presence of fraudulent entities and self-serving individuals requires public vigilance and informed giving.

The grand illusion of change accompanying powerful documentaries and movements must be met with the sobering reality that meaningful progress often requires more than financial contributions. It necessitates a collective commitment to ensuring that charities and nonprofit organizations operate with integrity, that funds are used effectively, and that those in need are genuinely helped. In the pursuit of a better world, it is our collective responsibility to demand transparency and hold charitable organizations accountable for the promises they make.

Chapter 22

How Dishonest People Appear Honest

Dishonest individuals often appear trustworthy through psychological techniques and social behaviors. These strategies enable them to create an illusion of honesty that can be difficult to penetrate. As members of a society where deception is prevalent, we are all potential targets. Understanding these techniques is not just informative, but a necessary tool for self-protection.

CONFIDENCE AND CHARISMA

One of the most effective ways dishonest people gain trust is through confidence and charisma. They often speak with unwavering self-assurance, making their statements seem more credible. For instance, a con artist might confidently explain a complex investment scheme, making potential victims believe in its legitimacy simply because of their confident delivery.

Additionally, their charismatic presence can be disarming. Charismatic individuals are naturally likable and engaging, making it hard for others to believe they are lying. Consider a charming salesperson who uses their personality to sell a defective product. Their charisma makes it difficult for customers to suspect foul play, even when the product fails.

DETAIL AND CONSISTENCY

Another hallmark of a skilled deceiver is their ability to provide detailed and plausible stories.

Elaborate accounts can be more convincing than vague ones. For example, someone fabricating a job experience might give specific details about their daily tasks, colleagues, and projects, making their story more believable.

Consistency is also crucial. Dishonest individuals ensure their stories remain consistent over time, reducing suspicion. If questioned about past events, they recount the exact details each time, reinforcing their credibility. For example, someone lying about their whereabouts might meticulously remember the fabricated details to avoid slipping up.

EMOTIONAL MANIPULATON

Dishonest people are adept at emotional manipulation. They often display empathy and concern to make others feel understood and valued. This emotional connection lowers their targets' guards. For instance, a fraudulent charity organizer might express deep empathy for a cause, making donors feel like they are contributing to something meaningful.

Another common tactic is playing the victim. They garner sympathy and distract others from their dishonesty by presenting themselves as wronged or suffering. For example, an employee caught embezzling funds might claim financial hardship or personal crises to elicit sympathy and deflect attention from their crime.

BODY LANGUAGE AND MICRO-EXPRESSIONS

Controlled body language is another tool in the deceiver's arsenal. They maintain steady eye contact, open body language, and controlled facial expressions. These non-verbal cues are associated with honesty, making their deceit less detectable. A politician lying about a scandal might use confident gestures and direct eye contact to appear sincere.

Minimizing involuntary facial expressions, or micro-expressions, also helps. These brief, involuntary facial expressions can reveal genuine emotions. By mastering their micro-expressions, deceptive individuals maintain a facade of sincerity. For example, a poker player might control their micro-expressions to prevent opponents from reading their true intentions.

REPUTATION AND SOCIAL PROOF
Building a good reputation over time makes it harder for others to question a person's integrity. A solid reputation acts as a shield against accusations of dishonesty. For example, a long-time community leader involved in fraudulent activities might rely on their established reputation to deflect suspicion.

Social proof is another powerful tool. Surrounding themselves with people who vouch for their character reinforces their perceived honesty. A dishonest businessperson might have testimonials from seemingly credible sources, making it difficult for potential clients to doubt their trustworthiness.

SELECTIVE TRUTHS
Mixing truths with lies makes deceit more challenging to detect. Partial truths lend credibility to an overall story, making the lies more believable. For instance, someone lying about their qualifications might mix accurate details of their education with fabricated job experiences.

Another subtle tactic is omitting critical details rather than directly lying. This strategy makes dishonesty less obvious. For example, politicians might omit discussing controversial policies in their campaigns, presenting a selective and favorable image to the public.

GENUINE EMOTIONS

Dishonest individuals often practice displaying genuine emotions, making their deceit harder to spot. Practiced emotions appear authentic, adding credibility to their lies. For example, an actor convincingly portraying a charitable persona can deceive audiences into supporting their cause.

Another tactic is managing emotional responses to appear more sincere. Controlled emotions help maintain the illusion of honesty. For instance, a defendant in court might practice appearing remorseful to gain sympathy from the jury.

MIRRORING AND BUILDING RAPPORT

Adopting body language and speech patterns like another person builds rapport and trust. This technique makes others feel more connected to the deceiver. For example, a negotiator might mirror a client's posture and tone, creating a sense of camaraderie and trust.

Actively building relationships and trust further reduces suspicion. A dishonest person who invests time in forming genuine-seeming connections is less likely to be suspected. For example, a scam artist might build friendships with their target before exploiting that trust.

DEFLECTION AND REDIRECTION

Deflecting questions and concerns shifts focus away from dishonesty. This technique helps avoid scrutiny and challenging questions. For instance, a politician might deflect questions about a scandal by emphasizing unrelated achievements.

Redirecting conversations helps maintain control over the narrative. By steering discussions away from sensitive topics, deceivers prevent their deceit from being exposed. For example, a business leader accused of misconduct might redirect conversations to plans, avoiding detailed inquiries about past actions.

PREPARATION AND PRACTICE
Dishonest individuals often prepare and rehearse their lies, which makes their falsehoods more convincing and harder to detect. For example, a fraudulent job applicant might rehearse fabricated resume details to avoid inconsistencies during interviews.

Anticipating potential questions and having ready responses helps avoid being caught off guard. This foresight ensures their story remains consistent. For example, a student lying about cheating might anticipate possible questions from teachers and prepare plausible answers.

Understanding these techniques can help identify and deal with dishonest individuals more effectively. By recognizing the strategies used to create an illusion of honesty, we can better discern truth from deception. Armed with this knowledge, we can take control of our interactions and protect ourselves from being manipulated.

Chapter 23

The Struggle to Acknowledge Being Duped by an Organization

Realizing and admitting that an organization or charity has deceived one can be incredibly challenging. Several psychological and social factors contribute to this difficulty, creating significant barriers to facing the truth.

COGNITIVE DISSONANCE

Cognitive dissonance occurs when a person's beliefs conflict with reality. When individuals realize they have been deceived, it creates an uncomfortable mental conflict. To reduce this discomfort, they might rationalize their decisions, convincing themselves that they had valid reasons for supporting the organization. This rationalization process helps them maintain their belief system intact, even in the face of contradictory evidence. For example, a person might argue that their donations were still used for a good cause, even if the organization was dishonest.

SUNK COST FALLACY

The sunk cost fallacy is a powerful psychological phenomenon where people continue to invest in something because of the time, money, or effort they've already put into it rather than cutting their losses. In the context of being deceived by an organization, individuals might support it to justify their past investments. They may fear admitting their mistake would mean accepting their contributions were wasted. This fallacy often leads to a cycle of continued support, hoping to eventually see a return on their investment, even when evidence suggests otherwise.

IDENTITY AND EGO PROTECTION

Acknowledging deception can be perceived as a personal failure, challenging one's self-image and ego. Many individuals derive a sense of identity and pride from their charitable actions or affiliations with organizations. Admitting they were duped can lead to embarrassment, shame, or guilt, which are difficult emotions to confront. They might deny the deception or downplay its significance to protect their ego. This denial helps them preserve their self-esteem and avoid the discomfort of acknowledging their vulnerability.

SOCIAL PRESSURE

Social dynamics play a significant role in maintaining support for an organization. If individuals are part of a community that strongly supports the organization, admitting they were deceived can lead to social isolation or backlash. The fear of being ostracized or criticized by peers can be a powerful motivator to continue endorsing the organization. This social pressure can create an environment where dissenting voices are silenced, and individuals feel compelled to conform to the group's beliefs and actions.

HOPE AND OPTIMISM

Hope and optimism are natural human tendencies that can keep people invested in an organization despite evidence of deceit. Individuals often cling to believing their trust was not misplaced and that the organization will eventually fulfill its promises. Occasional positive outcomes or organizational reassurances can reinforce this hope. Individuals maintain their faith by focusing on these glimmers of hope and avoid confronting the harsh reality of being deceived.

MISINFORMATION AND DENIAL

Continuous exposure to misleading information from the organization can keep individuals in denial. Organizations adept at controlling narratives and disseminating misinformation can create an environment where accurate information is hard to access. This misinformation reinforces the belief in the organization's legitimacy and obscures the truth. Individuals might selectively interpret information to fit their beliefs, further entrenching their support and denial.

These psychological and social factors create a formidable barrier to acknowledging deception. Cognitive dissonance, the sunk cost fallacy, identity and ego protection, social pressure, hope and optimism, and misinformation all contribute to the difficulty of facing the truth. Understanding these dynamics is crucial for addressing and overcoming the challenges those duped face, paving the way for greater awareness and critical thinking in their future decisions.

Chapter 24

Unmasking PsyOps - The Art of Psychological Operations

In this chapter, we will delve into the intriguing world of psychological operations, commonly referred to as "PsyOps." These covert tactics are designed to manipulate and influence individuals or groups' thoughts, emotions, and behaviors. Throughout history, governments, intelligence agencies, and even non-state actors have harnessed the power of PsyOps to achieve a range of objectives, from swaying public opinion to achieving strategic military goals. Let's uncover the mysteries and strategies behind these psychological maneuvers.

WHAT ARE PSYCHOLOGICAL OPERATIONS?

Psychological operations, or PsyOps, represent a strategic communication process that aims to shape the perceptions and behaviors of a target audience. These target audiences can be as diverse as enemy combatants, domestic or international populations, or even one's own military forces. The primary goal of PsyOps is to achieve a specific outcome by influencing the psychology of the individuals or groups involved.

THE HISTORICAL ROOTS OF PSYOPS

PsyOps is not a recent development. Throughout history, militaries and governments have employed various forms of psychological warfare to manipulate their adversaries. Propaganda, deception, and misinformation have played a pivotal role in conflicts dating back to ancient times.

In contemporary warfare, psychological operations are employed alongside conventional military strategies. These operations weaken the enemy's resolve, demoralize their forces, and gain strategic advantages without engaging in direct combat. Remember, enemy in the former sentence is how the actors of psychological operations see their opponents/followers. The people on the other side of a PsyOp may see themselves as supporters of a cause, donors, fans, etc.

THE PSYCHOLOGICAL TOOLBOX

These tools include propaganda, disinformation, information warfare, and social media manipulation. Fear is the number one weapon employed against the masses. The number two is campaigns that herald a great cause, but never intend to meet the objective. This was huge in the medical freedom movement with the "goal" of reversing the 1986 provision that gave indemnity to the vaccine manufacturers, We will talk about that more soon. Understanding these tactics is essential for recognizing and guarding against manipulation in the modern information age.

The use of PsyOps raises essential ethical and legal questions. Is it justifiable to manipulate perceptions and beliefs, even if it serves a "more significant" strategic purpose? Who gets to ultimately decide what cause is worthy of using manipulation on the populace? Are people's freedoms taken into account when a PsyOp is planned? I venture to say the goal of a PsyOp is to strategically strip people of their freedoms while getting them to agree that the losses are somehow in their best interests. We see this type of campaign every time there is an act of violence in the world and politicians start calling for an end to second amendment rights, using magazine count and weapon specs to justify the need to strip citizens of their guns and ammunitions. PsyOps like the one I just mentioned are easy to see, but not all are so apparent, and that is precisely why the method is called a psychological operation. The battle is for the mind and stagnating action towards a cause or causing people to act in a specified manner that meets the goals and ends of the campaign.

COUNTERMEASURES AND RESILIENCE

Building psychological resilience and critical thinking skills is crucial in an age where information can be weaponized. You will gain insights into how to recognize and resist manipulative tactics, both in the context of warfare and in everyday life.

As we journey through the world of psychological operations, we will discover that PsyOps are not confined to the realm of covert military actions. The principles behind these operations are relevant in marketing, politics, and even personal relationships. Understanding PsyOps is a matter of defense and a tool for empowerment and informed decision-making in a world saturated with information and influence. I have made it my life's mission to raise proper awareness to the players and issues stuck on replay because the tactics work. There was a time I was under the spell of the medical freedom movement until I continued looking for results and had to concede that no movement was made towards the promises, just a lot of money raised towards goals that never had a plan of being actualized.

Chapter 25

The Evolution of Psychological Operations

Psychological Operations (PsyOps), also known as Psychological Warfare (PsyWar), have played a significant role in military and political conflict history. This chapter delves into the history, evolution, and a comprehensive explanation of PsyOps, shedding light on how this form of warfare has influenced perceptions, attitudes, and behavior.

THE ORIGINS OF PSYOPS

Psychological operations have their roots in ancient warfare and have evolved significantly over the centuries. The use of psychological tactics to manipulate the minds of adversaries can be traced back to Sun Tzu's "The Art of War" in ancient China. Sun Tzu emphasized the importance of deception and manipulating the enemy's perception as essential elements of successful warfare. However, modern PsyOps techniques began to take shape during the 20th century, particularly during World War I and World War II.

WORLD WAR I AND WORLD WAR II

During World War I, both the Allied and Central Powers engaged in various propaganda campaigns to boost morale, gather support, and weaken the enemy's resolve. These efforts included distributing leaflets, creating posters, and disseminating news through various media outlets. Notable examples include the British propaganda efforts to depict the

Germans as inhumane aggressors and the Germans' counter-propaganda campaign.

World War II witnessed a significant expansion of psychological operations. The United States established the Office of Strategic Services (OSS), responsible for conducting various covert and psychological warfare activities. The British used their expertise in deception, most famously in Operation Fortitude, which misled the Germans about the location of the D-Day landings.

THE COLD WAR ERA

The Cold War era marked a period of intense competition between the United States and the Soviet Union. PSYOPS played a crucial role in shaping global perceptions and opinions. Both superpowers engaged in propaganda warfare, spreading their ideologies and attempting to influence nations worldwide. Radio Free Europe and Radio Liberty were established by the United States to broadcast anti-communist messages into Eastern Europe. At the same time, the Soviets used Radio Moscow and other outlets to promote their ideology.

MODERN PSYOPS

The end of the Cold War did not diminish the importance of psychological operations. Instead, it led to the development of more sophisticated and subtle tactics. PsyOps became integral to modern warfare, counterterrorism efforts, and diplomacy. The 21st century witnessed the widespread use of social media and information warfare, which further expanded the realm of psychological operations.

THE ROLE OF PSYOPS TODAY

Modern psychological operations encompass a broad spectrum of activities, including propaganda, public affairs, and civil affairs. These operations are conducted by military and civilian agencies and can target both domestic and international audiences. The digital age has opened new avenues for influencing perceptions, such as social media campaigns, disinformation, and cyber warfare.

KEY PRINCIPLES OF PSYOPS

Understand the Target Audience: Effective psychological operations require a deep understanding of the cultural, social, and psychological factors that shape the perceptions and behavior of the target audience. This is where controlled opposition will come in. "Leaders" are planted in movements to gain the trust and backing of the group being infiltrated.

1. Credibility: The source of the information and messaging is critical. It must be credible to the audience to have any influence.

2. Coordinated Efforts: Successful PsyOps involve coordination between military, intelligence, and diplomatic agencies to ensure a cohesive strategy.

3. Ethical Considerations: The ethical implications of psychological operations are essential, as the use of deceptive tactics can raise ethical concerns.

Psychological operations have come a long way since their ancient origins, evolving alongside technological advancements and changes in global politics. In the 21st century, PSYOPS continue to be a vital and often hostile component of military and diplomatic strategies, shaping how nations conduct themselves worldwide. Understanding the history and principles of psychological operations is crucial for military professionals and civilians in an era where information and perception hold significant power.

Chapter 26

Medical Psychological Operations (Medical PsyOps)

Medical Psychological Operations, often called Medical PsyOps, represent a unique and complex subset of psychological operations. While traditional PsyOps focus on influencing perceptions, attitudes, and behaviors in the context of military and political conflict, Medical PSYOPS have a distinct humanitarian and medical mission.

THE EMERGENCE OF MEDICAL PSYOPS
Medical PsyOps have evolved in response to the changing nature of warfare and the increasing importance of winning hearts and minds, both on the battlefield and in post-conflict reconstruction. The concept of using medical care as a psychological weapon emerged in the mid-20th century, gaining prominence during the Vietnam War.

During the Vietnam War, the United States implemented Medical PSYOPS through the Civilian Irregular Defense Group (CIDG) program. This initiative provided medical and humanitarian assistance to local populations, helping to foster trust and cooperation while undermining support for the Viet Cong.

PRINCIPLES OF MEDICAL PSYOPS
Humanitarian Mission: Medical PsyOps prioritize humanitarian care as their primary goal. This includes providing medical assistance, training local

healthcare workers, and supporting healthcare infrastructure.

Hearts and Minds: The fundamental objective of Medical PsyOps is to build trust and goodwill with local populations by providing much-needed medical services. This engenders positive perceptions and cooperation.

Strategic Messaging: Information and messaging are essential components of Medical PsyOps. Communication strategies should emphasize the benevolent intentions of the medical teams and the willingness to help those in need.

Cultural Sensitivity: Understanding and respecting the cultural norms and beliefs of the local population is crucial to the success of Medical PsyOps. Adherence to cultural norms helps build trust.

MODERN APPLICATIONS

Medical PsyOps have been applied in various military and humanitarian missions in the 21st century:

- Military Operations: In conflict zones like Afghanistan and Iraq, military medical teams have provided care to local civilians, including surgeries, vaccinations, and basic healthcare. These efforts aim to foster cooperation and mitigate hostilities.

- Disaster Relief: Medical PsyOps principles have been applied in disaster relief operations worldwide, where medical teams provide aid to disaster-affected populations.

This builds goodwill and enhances international cooperation.

- ➤ Counterterrorism: In counterterrorism efforts, the provision of medical aid to communities affected by extremist ideologies can help reduce support for radical groups. It can also serve as a counter-narrative against extremist propaganda.

- ➤ Diplomacy and Soft Power: Medical PsyOps are not limited to military contexts. They are also a diplomatic tool to strengthen international relations and soft power. Nations can project a positive image globally by providing medical assistance and expertise.

ETHICAL CONSIDERATIONS

Medical PsyOps, like other forms of psychological operations, raise ethical concerns. One of the primary ethical considerations is the potential exploitation of medical care for strategic or political objectives. The medical community must adhere to strict ethical guidelines to ensure patient care is never compromised for strategic gain.

Medical Psychological Operations represent an innovative approach to humanitarian assistance, military cooperation, and diplomacy. By emphasizing the delivery of medical care and establishing trust, these operations have proven effective in fostering goodwill and cooperation in complex, often hostile, environments. Ethical considerations remain paramount, ensuring that medical care is never compromised for strategic or political objectives. In an era where the humanitarian and strategic aspects of the conflict are intertwined, Medical PsyOps have become a critical tool in the toolbox of military and humanitarian organizations.

A current example of a medical PsyOp that invaded every sector of our lives from the economy to religious organizations to government, to how we behaved, bought things, etc. would be the shutdown of 2020 that is still having lasting negative impact globally. We could go more in depth on this topic, but that's its own book and discussion outside the scope of this work. I am referencing it to show that the medical freedom movement is a small Medical PsyOp compared to what was pulled off globally.

Chapter 27

Hollywood IS the Propaganda Machine

Before delving into Del Bigtree's role, it's crucial to grasp that Hollywood frequently collaborates with government agencies and influences public perception. It's not just entertainment; it's a strategic arm of psychological operations.

In a very important essay that ran in March of 2017 in <u>The American Journal of Economics and Sociology</u>, Pearse Redmond goes into great detail about the "conspiracy" between governmental agencies and Hollywood. His essay, titled "The Historical Roots of CIA-Hollywood Propaganda" goes into great detail about the use of this symbiotic relationship starting in 1915, during the First World War. While I won't go into great detail about the specific war machine that this relationship yields, I would like to share some of his writing that is relevant to understanding what I'm getting at here:

> Propaganda also uses popular media as a means of manipulating and controlling domestic populations...In order to maintain popular support and a patriotic spirit, government agencies have also made use of popular media. In particular, they have used Hollywood as the premier vehicle with which to propagandize the populace...The CIA and Pentagon are the two most powerful institutions engaged in

> this form of propaganda in Hollywood. They have developed tactics and an overarching strategy over many years, perfecting it to a near science (281-282).

Redmond goes on to say that to combat this issue, we must understand how it works, which is what the entirety of his essay continues to do. I happen to agree with his premise. His essay deals with very specific example of this mind warfare, but his premise applies to the warfare transmitted on the ideals, social norms, and opinions of the American people.

His conclusion mirrors my sentiments as well:

> This situation raises a number of questions and realities that we need to seriously address. Is this something that we as a society want to ignore and allow? Letting the government and its military and intelligence arms dictate what we view as entertainment is a dangerous road to go down. This helps maintain the constant state of warfare that we are in...The state is making us complicit as a population in its crimes. This allows for it to continue on its present course and strive to go even further...(307).

The fight for our medical freedom has been and continues to be a war, especially when there are permanent casualties involved. This leaves anyone on the public stage open for scrutiny as those of us who would preserve ourselves from being acted upon delve into the available information to make informed decisions for ourselves and the people we love.

Before I go any further, I want to put a personal disclaimer here. In doing research for this book, I also looked up the public figure libel law since some of the names that will show up in the subsequent pages are sue happy. I am happy to report that nothing forthcoming meets the standard of the libel law which states that "to win a libel suit, a public figure must prove the publisher of the false statements acted with actual malice. Actual malice means that the publisher knew that the statements were false or acted with reckless disregard for whether they were true or false." My research is solid, and I encourage each of you to do your own research and form your own conclusions.

Nothing in this book is malicious, it is borne out of concern and intense observation to protect those I care about. As I stated earlier, I was a huge fan of the players in this movement until I realized that their promises were material misrepresentations of their motive. They made grand sweeping promises to their fans that never materialized and therefore should be held accountable for misrepresentations that led to huge financial donor turnout. This is my attempt to right my wrongs of public support for a group of people that have not followed up on their initial guarantees.

CATCHING THE DISSENTERS

Controlled opposition operates within a carefully orchestrated plan – to capture individuals who question the mainstream media's narrative on C-19 but haven't delved deep into the intricacies. These people retain some faith in vaccines but are hesitant about the new experimental C-19 vaccines. To combat any dissent a very nefarious plot was enacted. It is smoke and mirrors of controlled opposition coming out against the agenda and then starting to make a mockery of it.

There were a lot of social media influencers that made their way onto television and interviews by the tactic of flip-flopping on their former "anti-vaccine" viewpoints. The switch was believable because the social media influencers that gained public audiences seemed to be unknowns before their breakout roles. Looking further into them, they had acting backgrounds and were very open about that. Sadly, many people didn't blink an eye at that tidbit. While the examples at the forefront of my mind do not warrant being named, their switching of sides was used to gaslight those that held firm. The headlines heralded "former anti-vaxxers" that received the vaccine as trailblazers for others to stop "denying the science." If you followed the social media influencers past the videos of them being jabbed, you would see gaslighting videos making fun of people not getting the shot intermittent with health issues and emergency hospital visits while still saying they would rather have health issues than be dead from the C-19 virus.

At this juncture, I would just like to point out that most of us that have not had the shot are still alive and have no adverse effects from the vaccine, so that is a moot point. This argument is akin to the childhood vaccine schedule supporters who say they would rather have an autistic child than a dead child. To that I say, while I love my two autistic vaccine injured children, I still mourn for the normal lives they will never lead. Autism is its own death. We should all be careful what we say.

THE ILLUSION OF ANTI-VACCINE OPPOSITION

The strategy involves creating a facade of anti-vaccine opposition. It seeks to draw in these individuals, temper their dissent, and channel their skepticism into a controlled, manufactured movement. This movement, however, is never allowed to become too radical or extreme.

Behind this charade stand influential players – Big Pharma, the banking elite, and clandestine government agencies. They understand that they must maintain control over the opposition's narrative to further their agendas. Allowing dissenters to wander off and conduct their research is not an option, so the research is presented by paid actors. We will talk about the recorded revenue jumps for the organizations headed by our key players shortly.

To achieve this, they construct an artificial pen with boundaries defining what constitutes acceptable dissent. This controlled space prevents individuals from asking more profound questions about viruses and vaccines, effectively boxing them in.

This new pen is the destination they intend for everyone. They craft an exaggerated, villainous narrative to lure the dissenters, featuring figures like Fauci, Gates, and Pfizer. Over time, they unveil this illusion, making the new pen appear more appealing than the mainstream. It becomes acceptable to question and attack the narratives created by the faux enemies like Fauci, Gates, and pharmaceutical companies while also reporting on the virus in a way that spreads fear and builds a question in the mind of weaker followers: "Can I risk a brush with a deadly virus as explained by my favorite voice on the subject?. Or should I line up to avoid the virus by getting the vaccine?" From the accounts of some of the people that have reached out to me, they opted for the latter option after hearing specific things about C19 from one of the controlled opposition speakers.

SHEEPHERDERS LEADING THE FLOCK

To steer the dissenters into this controlled pen, they need leaders, or rather, puppet shepherds. These individuals, like Del Bigtree, are tasked with gathering the strays and skeptics, guiding them into the new fake opposition. To understand how intelligent people that question the official narrative can be fooled, I need to explain another level of the propaganda machine.

LIMITED HANGOUT OPERATION

Del's role mirrors a limited hangout operation. A morsel of truth is unveiled – vaccines can be dangerous. Yet, this morsel is swiftly shrouded in layers of deception – we can make vaccines safer – and misdirection, guiding the narrative back into controlled territory. Followers may disagree initially but the dissent morphs from a firm "NO" to "Well, if they were safer I would like the added layer of protection from illness" to "Who wouldn't want a defense system that keeps them from downtime from being sick—no missed school or work or play. Yeah, that would be great, let's move the theory to reality." Suddenly, the firm no has become an issue where if the sheepherder would profess a safe way, the follower would take the bait.

WHERE DOES BIGTREE FIT IN?

While many perceive Del as a champion battling corruption, a closer examination reveals a different story. We must scrutinize Del's career and role in this elaborate charade to truly understand this hypothesis. The availability of an IMBD page that shows a less than stellar performance in prior attempts to stardom shows a hunger for the limelight, at least. His work as producer of "The Doctors" raises questions of his missing anti-vaccine status while making that show.

    Stardom was achieved when he reached a radically underserved population of parents of vaccine damaged children who were waiting for someone to herald the cause. This hidden population had started making noise online and finding one another to raise a collective cry against the childhood vaccine agenda and then VIOLA, we were handed a cause pretending to be a movement and leaders making promises like an overturn to the 1986 Indemnity clause that kept vaccine manufacturers from being sued for faulty products. This happened despite the Supreme Court ruling that vaccines are unavoidably unsafe, which is now heavily censored online, though we will get there in the next book to make sure our bases are covered. Next though, I would like to cover some medical research that should be common knowledge among the medical freedom movement. If someone isn't aware, the information is available, and if you are, it's a refresher.

Chapter 28

The Art of Grifting – A Cynical Exploitation

THE CON ARTIST'S SYMPHONY

Grifting, the age-old art of deception and manipulation, is a symphony of chicanery orchestrated by the most cunning individuals in society. It's a dark and intricate craft, weaving complex webs of falsehoods and preying upon the trust of unsuspecting victims. In the world of grifting, there are no virtuosos, only maestros of malevolence, conducting their fraudulent orchestra with expertise honed over time. You have most likely heard the old adage that "the best lies contain a shred of truth." The issue arises when we have to discern between the shred of truth, "medical freedom and bodily autonomy are important in the face of making medical decisions that can only be made by an individual and their family," versus stripping out promises made that will be unkept (future faking) to raise funds immediately for a utopian cause.

THE ENABLERS OF GRIFT

Every successful con artist needs an audience to perform their acts of deception, and the grifters of the modern age have found a vast and receptive audience in the digital realm. They expertly exploit the gullibility of those who yearn for sensational narratives and seek affirmation over information. With the advent of social media, these grifters have found a sprawling stage where they can perform their deceptions to an audience that's not only eager but also ravenous for conspiracies and quick solutions to complex issues.

Now, let's delve into the vaccine grifters, a specific breed of con artists who have mastered the art of exploiting public concerns about vaccines. They seize upon genuine fears and manipulate narratives to fit their ulterior motives. These grifters often employ charisma, cherry-picked evidence, and pseudoscience to build cult-like followings, where skepticism turns into unquestioning devotion. The cherry-picked information conceals their ultimate agenda—"safer" vaccines of which their cohorts hold patents.

THE TANGLED WEB OF DECEPTION

Grifting, in the context of vaccine hesitancy, involves the meticulous crafting of narratives designed to prey on public opinion. It thrives on the erosion of trust in scientific consensus and government institutions, which is an absolute certainty for the Medical Freedom Movement, and rightfully so. The grifters spin tales of "hidden truths" and "suppressed evidence," luring vulnerable individuals into their intricate web of deception, where they become unwitting actors in a grand theatrical production. These grifters also claim to be the ones breaking the information to protect people and make themselves into the likeness of a savior to the masses. More money will allow them to bring more information forward. It's a cyclical scheme that many have fallen into. You will see the extent when we look at the numbers.

MONETIZING MISINFORMATION

In the age of the internet, misinformation isn't just a byproduct of grifting; it's a thriving and highly lucrative business. Grifters amass enormous fortunes by peddling books, videos, supplements, and exclusive membership programs that promise to "unlock the secrets" or "reveal the cover-ups." Their income flows directly from the pockets of those desperately seeking answers, regardless of whether those answers are based on facts or fabrications.

THE CONSEQUENCES OF GRIFTING

The consequences of grifting are far-reaching, extending well beyond the deceptive narratives spun by grifters. Fighting grifting in the Medical Freedom Movement is akin to battling an ever-evolving hydra. The battle will endure as long as individuals are willing to believe in the elaborate tales spun by grifters. However, the key to combating grifting lies in education, critical thinking, and promoting trust in reputable sources. It's a battle of minds and morals, where the ultimate victory is restoring truth and safeguarding public health.

Grifting is not merely a shady endeavor but a dark and malevolent art form, cynically exploiting human vulnerability for personal gain. In the world of vaccine hesitancy, grifters sow falsehoods for profit, leaving behind a trail of misinformation and shattered trust. The ongoing battle against grifting is a test of society's resilience against manipulation. Still, with knowledge, discernment, and unwavering commitment to truth, we can hope to unmask the charlatans and protect advocates from their insidious deceptions.

Chapter 29

Non-Profits: The Manipulation of Social Good

Once heralded as fortresses of altruism and social betterment, non-profit organizations have, in many cases, transformed into the subtle but effective tools of the ruling class. Beneath the veneer of charitable endeavors and noble missions lies a web of influence and control that perpetuates the status quo and consolidates power in the hands of the elite.

THE FAÇADE OF ALTRUISM
The origins of non-profits as instruments of societal change are rooted in admirable intentions. These organizations were designed to serve as a vehicle for societal betterment, to address pressing issues, and to provide a helping hand to those in need. However, their evolution tells a different story.

With its vast wealth and resources, the ruling class recognized the potential of non-profits early on. They co-opted the non-profit sector, bending it to their will and transforming it into a mechanism that serves their interests rather than the greater good. The tax-exempt status granted to non-profits became a powerful tool for the ruling class to consolidate their wealth while appearing philanthropic.

CHARITY BEGINS (AND ENDS) AT THE TOP
Follow the money, and you'll find that a significant portion of charitable donations from the ruling class flows right back into their own spheres of

influence. Museums, operas, art galleries, elite universities, private hospitals, and family foundations are the primary beneficiaries of this largesse. These institutions cater to the elite, perpetuating their cultural hegemony and social standing.

PUPPETEERS OF CHANGE

Non-profits should be driven by their mission to bring about social change and address systemic issues. However, many of these organizations have become manipulated marionettes. A substantial portion of their funding comes from charitable foundations and direct donations by individuals who influence and control society's levers.

In a cruel irony, non-profits serving the most vulnerable, those at the base of the socioeconomic pyramid, often find themselves beholden to the whims and guidelines set by the ruling class. Their efforts become a never-ending quest for approval and funding, a process that shackles them to the status quo.

THE MIRAGE OF SOCIAL SERVICES AND CHANGE

One of the most insidious aspects of this manipulation is the redirection of non-profit efforts toward social services. While these services are undoubtedly necessary, they often serve to uphold the status quo rather than oppose it. With its insatiable desire for control, the ruling class funds non-profit programming that fills gaps in service provision, extending outreach to underserved groups, all while emphasizing collaboration.

This strategic approach ensures that the ruling class remains in power and as the perceived savior of the masses. They keep hope alive but in a manner that perpetuates the very inequalities they claim to alleviate.

UNMASKING THE CHARADE

The current role of non-profits in our society must be exposed. It's imperative to question the motivations behind charitable donations and scrutinize the agendas that steer these organizations. We hope to break free from the clutches of the ruling class and strive for a society where social good prevails over self-interest only through transparency, critical analysis, and a reimagining of the non-profit sector.

Monetizing Misery

Chapter 30

Billionaire "Philanthropists" and the Swaying of Medical Information: The Case of Bill and Melinda Gates

Few names are as influential in global health as Bill and Melinda Gates. Through the Bill & Melinda Gates Foundation, they have poured billions of dollars into vaccine programs, particularly in third-world countries. While they present themselves as benevolent philanthropists, their actions and statements raise significant concerns about the ethical implications of their influence on medical information and public health policies.

THE GATES' ADVOCACY FOR VACCINES

Bill and Melinda Gates have been vocal advocates for vaccines, funding extensive immunization programs worldwide. Their foundation has partnered with various organizations, including the World Health Organization (WHO) and Gavi, the Vaccine Alliance, to promote vaccination to solve global health crises. Their efforts are particularly focused on third-world countries, where they argue vaccines can drastically reduce disease prevalence and improve health outcomes.

POPULATION CONTROL STATEMENTS

One of the most controversial aspects of Gates' advocacy is their public statements linking vaccine success to population control. Bill Gates has been quoted saying that with successful vaccination, among other health interventions, population growth could be curtailed. Critics have interpreted this statement as an indication of a hidden agenda to reduce population numbers through vaccination programs.

LEGAL AND ETHICAL CONCERNS

While the Gates Foundation does not explicitly impersonate doctors, its significant influence over global health policies and direct involvement in medical interventions raise ethical and legal questions. According to federal law, specifically 18 U.S. Code § 912, impersonating a doctor or giving medical advice without a license is illegal. This law is intended to protect individuals from unqualified persons making critical health decisions or providing medical care.

Although Bill and Melinda Gates do not directly administer vaccines, their foundation's funding and influence shape global health policies and practices. The concern lies in the potential for their directives to override local health authorities and experts, leading to a form of medical imperialism where their vision dictates healthcare outcomes in vulnerable regions.

THEIR WORK OVERSEAS

The Gates Foundation's work overseas is extensive and highly publicized. It has funded polio eradication efforts, malaria prevention programs, and widespread vaccination campaigns against diseases like measles and rotavirus. Its initiatives often involve large-scale immunization drives, educational campaigns, and the establishment of healthcare infrastructure in underdeveloped areas.

However, these programs have been subject to controversy. In some instances, their vaccination campaigns have faced resistance from local populations, who view them with suspicion and concern. There have been reports of adverse reactions to vaccines, and some communities have expressed fears about the long-term impacts of these immunization efforts.

INFLUENCE ON MEDICAL INFORMATION

The Gates' extensive financial contributions give them substantial leverage over global health organizations and initiatives. This influence extends to research funding, policy recommendations, and the dissemination of medical information. Critics argue that this concentration of power in the hands of a few individuals undermines democratic decision-making processes in public health and skews priorities towards the interests of wealthy donors rather than those of the affected populations.

Bill and Melinda Gates present their philanthropic efforts as altruistic contributions to global health. However, their significant influence over medical information and public health policies and controversial statements on population control raise critical ethical and legal questions. While their foundation has undoubtedly contributed to health improvements in many regions, the broader implications of their control over vaccine advocacy and implementation cannot be ignored. As influential figures in the health sector, their actions must be scrutinized to ensure that public health policies remain transparent, ethical, and aligned with the best interests of the populations they aim to serve.

Monetizing Misery

Chapter 31

Follow the Money – The Lucrative Pandemic-Fueled Windfall for Alleged 'Anti-Vaccination' Groups

THE BIRTH OF ADVOCACY GROUPS

In the wake of California's Senate Bill 277 (SB277) and its stringent vaccination requirements, the landscape of vaccine advocacy underwent a notable transformation. A new breed of advocacy groups emerged, fueled by the fervor of those opposed to vaccine mandates. Among them, the Informed Consent Action Network (ICAN), founded in 2016, and Robert F. Kennedy Jr.'s Children's Health Defense (CHD), (built from World Mercury Project in 2011) in 2018, stood out. Founded post-SB277, these organizations positioned themselves as voices of dissent in the vaccination discourse.

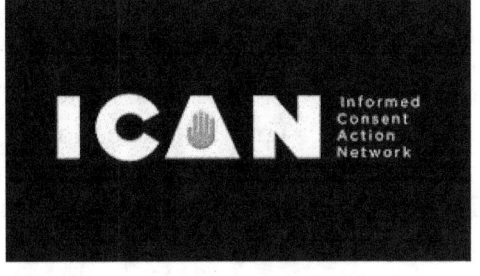

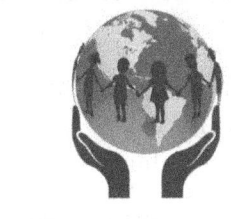

Fast forward to the unprecedented COVID-19 pandemic in 2020. As the world experienced a global health crisis, these anti-vaccination groups, ICAN and CHD, found themselves in a rather unexpected situation. Investigative reports by mainstream media outlets, such as NBC News, revealed a startling surge in donations to these groups during the pandemic year.

EYE-OPENING 2020 TAX RECORDS

In 2019, ICAN reported revenues of $437,918. However, an astonishing financial windfall occurred in 2020, as their revenue skyrocketed to a staggering $1.4 million, more than tripling their income. Then, in the last reportable year of 2022, it soared even further to $13.4 million, an increase of 2,960%. For CHD, the economic growth was similarly astounding. In 2019, CHD reported revenues of $223,223, but by 2020, their financial inflow had surged to an astonishing $2.4 million. Similarly, in the last reportable year of 2022, CHD's income soared to $23.5 million, which is an increase of 10,428%. Where did all this revenue come from? That's a question that must be asked under these circumstances. I personally believe this increase isn't from $25 donations. They refuse to name their donors, is it because pharma companies are at the top of the list? Inquiring minds want to know.

These revelations led to a deeper examination of the post-SB277 landscape. Advocacy groups that had once rallied against SB277 had now expanded their focus to include broader anti-vaccination campaigns. The financial backing they received during the pandemic raised questions about their influence and the motivations of their donors. Not only were the smaller financial donations rolling in but there are six-figure donations that should raise some eyebrows.

The pandemic had thrust these organizations into the spotlight, once again. Much like other non-degreed world stage actors making grand sweeping and loud medical statements to sway public opinion, the Medical Freedom Movement has very loud voices sans medical degrees presenting themselves as medical authorities on life and death topics, like what to take and not take medically. While not all of it is disagreeable, calling for the silencing of people like Bill Gates, who has no medical degree, comes off as hypocritical by the Medical Freedom Movement's non-degreed medical advice crowd.

The financial windfall experienced by anti-vaccination groups like ICAN and CHD during the COVID-19 pandemic underscored the evolving dynamics of vaccine advocacy. It also raised questions about the role of financial backing in shaping public health discourse. You can see their updated tax information below.

Monetizing Misery

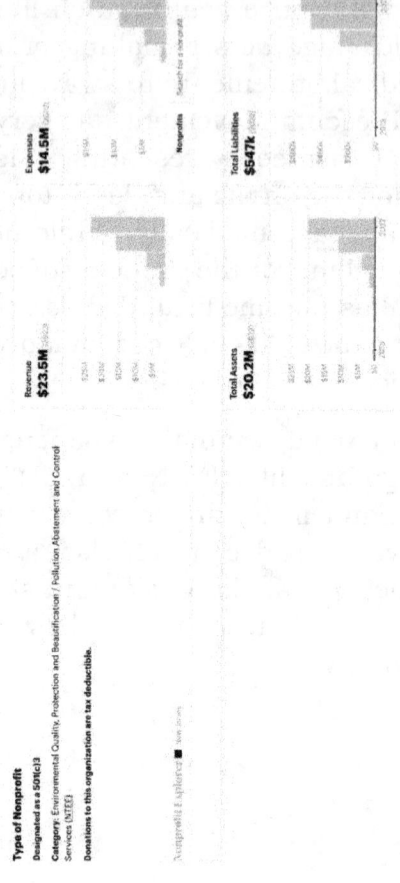

GregWyatt.com

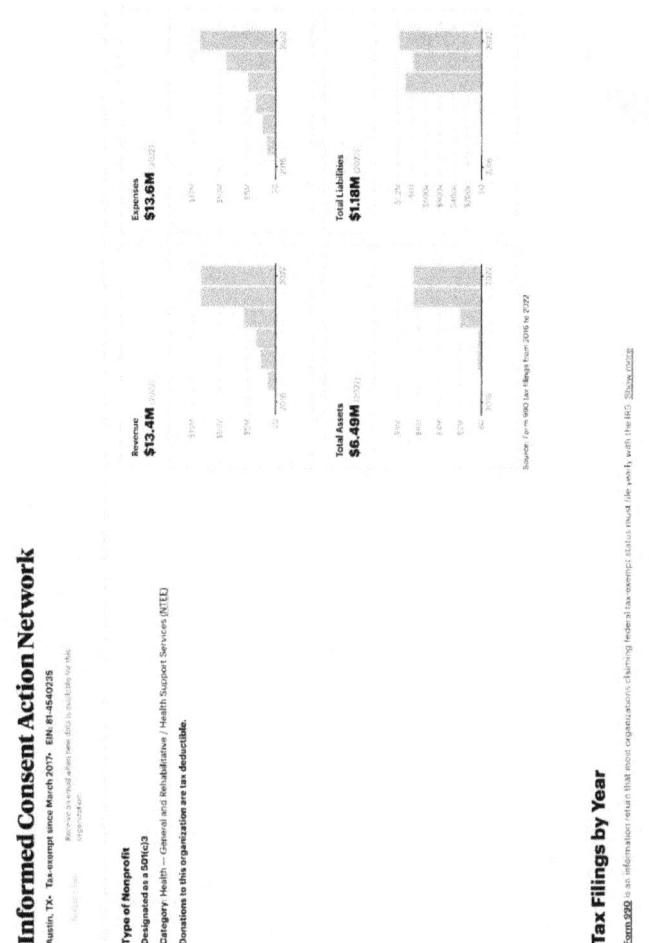

My question is: Are all of these millions from parents making donations? Or could it be pharmaceutical companies "donating" to keep the messaging watered down? There has been no movement to remove the 1986 Act, just lip service. There is always enough in the message to get people to give or believe in the organizations because most people don't go check the (non-existent) progress.

Chapter 32

VaxXed Revisited

Upon revisiting the film, previously unnoticed details now demand attention, prompting a closer examination of their implications. The narrative tactfully avoids directly implicating vaccines in the devastation wrought by the pandemic, instead focusing on the discourse of vaccine safety.

The unsettling reality emerges through Del Bigtree's advocacy: the genuine discourse on vaccine dangers has regressed by over two decades. The stark truth obscured by this regression is that vaccines are not the benign solutions they're portrayed to be; they exact a toll of death and injury.

The film's persistent labeling of the affliction as autism belies a deeper reality—it's not merely autism, but the result of chemical poisoning. Autism serves as a convenient euphemism, masking the true nature of the affliction.

At a pivotal moment, the film implicates the thimerosal-containing MMR vaccine in autism cases. This narrative serves Wakefield's vested interests, intertwined with a potential windfall. The exact financial implications notwithstanding, the conflict of interest looms large.

Brian Hooker's prominent role in the narrative draws attention, his personal connection lending credence to his assertions. Yet, his involvement in the charade raises questions about his true motivations and allegiances.

His intimate knowledge of vaccine injuries and the broader deceit surrounding viral narratives begs the question: is he complicit in perpetuating the deception?

The film's portrayal of clandestine meetings, coupled with the insinuation of a life of leisure awaiting those who orchestrate the grand scheme, lends credence to the notion of a hidden agenda at play.

The synchronicity between the birth of Hooker's son and pivotal moments in the narrative raises eyebrows, hinting at deeper connections and motivations.

As I wade through the remainder of the film, I'm acutely aware of the arduous task ahead, confronting the uncomfortable truths lurking within. A disquieting realization begins to take shape: the film's narrative appears crafted in collaboration with powerful entities— the CDC and perhaps even the clandestine hand of the CIA.

I urge you to invest the ninety minutes required to scrutinize this film, for within its frames lies a critical understanding of the shadows enveloping our reality. May our journey into this darkness be illuminated by discernment and unwavering resolve.

GregWyatt.com

Monetizing Misery

SECTION THREE:

Scientology in the Health Freedom Movement

Chapter 33

The Sinister Alliance: Scientology and the Health Freedom Movement

In the murky depths of the Health Freedom Movement lies a web of deception, manipulation, and exploitation. Among its ranks lurks a notorious figure, Scientology, a behemoth of a religious cult infamous for its insidious tactics and voracious appetite for control. Yet, Scientology's unholy alliance with the Health Freedom Movement exposes a darker truth—a truth that ensnares the vulnerable, preys on the desperate, and distorts reality.

At its core, the Health Freedom Movement promises solace to the lonely, purpose to the lost, and community to the isolated as families navigate the realities of v-injured family members requiring different levels of care. But beneath its façade of altruism lies a sinister agenda—a mission not of empowerment but of enslavement, not of enlightenment but of manipulation. It is a seduction of the mind, a journey into darkness disguised as a beacon of hope.

Scientology finds fertile ground to sow the seeds of its malevolent doctrine in this unholy union. It exploits the longing for belonging, the yearning for purpose, and the desperation for change with cunning precision. Under the guise of enlightenment, Scientology peddles false prophets and twisted truths, luring unsuspecting souls into its nefarious grasp.

But Scientology is not alone in its machinations. Alongside it, Christianity, once a bastion of faith and virtue, now stands accused of prostituting its sacred teachings for profit and power. False prophets, adorned in robes of righteousness, twist the scriptures to fit their narrative of greed and exploitation. "Send us money and believe, and you will receive," they proclaim, echoing the sinister refrain of their Scientology counterparts.

In this unholy trinity of deceit—Scientology, Christianity, and the Health Freedom Movement—the lines between faith and fraud blur, and the boundaries of reality bend to the will of the manipulators. Money flows like a river, filling the coffers of the cunning and draining the pockets of the faithful. Yet, in this grand illusion of enlightenment, common sense is sacrificed at the altar of deception, and truth becomes a casualty of the war for control.

As the shadows lengthen and the whispers of deceit grow louder, the true nature of this unholy alliance comes into focus. It is a pact forged in darkness, a covenant of manipulation, and a conspiracy of exploitation. And in its grip, the minds of the vulnerable are entangled, their dreams twisted, and their faith betrayed. While my place in exposing the players isn't popular, I will still be a watchman on a hill heralding the truth for those with eyes to see and ears to hear.

In the depths of the Health Freedom Movement, danger lurks unseen, and the seduction of the mind is a prelude to a darker fate. The illusionary concern is merely a money grab, and it works. All you have to do is look up the main "Health Freedom Movement" organizations headed by Bigtree and Kennedy and see headlines proclaiming the millions they have stolen from those in need while delivering nothing but headlines. In this section, we will examine how Scientology merges with the Health Freedom Movement.

Chapter 34

The Digital Web: Decoding Internet Addresses and the Shadowy Connections

In the depths of cyberspace, every click, every keystroke, leaves a digital footprint—a traceable path that winds its way through the vast expanse of the internet. At the heart of this digital realm lies the mysterious infrastructure of internet addresses, the invisible lines that connect users to websites, servers, and networks, creating webs within the Web. Understanding how these addresses work unveils a world of hidden connections, undercover alliances, and alarming implications.

Internet addresses, often called IP addresses, are virtual coordinates that guide data packets to their intended destinations. Each device connected to the internet, whether a computer, smartphone, or server, is assigned a unique IP address, much like a street address in the physical world. These addresses are organized into ranges, allocated by regional internet registries and internet service providers, ensuring seamless communication across the global network.

The alarming prospect of inadvertently linking a health freedom-associated domain to a specific IP address range raises unsettling questions about the integrity of the digital landscape. Such a scenario suggests a deliberate manipulation of internet infrastructure—a covert attempt to obscure online content's origins and subvert the principles of transparency and accountability.

Delving deeper into this digital mystery reveals a tangled web. The names Del Bigtree and Lori Jean Raines emerge as key players in this shadowy drama, their connections to Texas community organizing and Scientology casting a pall of suspicion over their actions. Raines, renowned for her involvement in the "Texas Million's March," shares ties with Jonathan Lockwood, an undercover Scientologist whose influence extends into political lobbying and advocacy.

The emergence of the "National Movement of Concerned Citizens," a purported protest coalition with dubious origins, further complicates the narrative. Analysis of this coalition suggests a convergence of interests between Scientology and certain government agencies, raising concerns about the extent of their influence and the agendas they seek to advance. Could Del Bigtree, with his connections to the U.S. Department of State, be acting as a conduit for Scientology within the corridors of power?

The implications are profound and far-reaching. The convergence of digital manipulation, political maneuvering, and ideological fervor paints a troubling picture of a world where information is weaponized, dissent is silenced, and truth becomes a casualty of the digital age. In other words, it is the perfect setup for monetizing misery.

As we peel back the layers of this digital tapestry, one thing becomes clear: the need for vigilance, transparency, and accountability has never been greater. For in the shadows of cyberspace, unseen forces wield immense power.

SECTION FOUR:

Why the Tactics Work

Monetizing Misery

Chapter 35

The Struggle of Cognitive Dissonance

WHEN FOOD IS MORE THAN FUEL

Imagine you've spent the better part of your life adhering to a particular dietary regimen—a diet you've come to believe is healthy and morally superior. Let's call it the "Veggie Vitality" diet. This diet has shaped your identity; it's what you proudly proclaim to friends and family. You've extolled its virtues, arguing passionately about the benefits for your health and the planet.

You've thrived on your Veggie Vitality diet, taking pride in your food choices and sharing your enthusiasm with others. Your refrigerator is filled with vibrant vegetables, plant-based proteins, and dairy alternatives. You've been an advocate, even joining local groups and forums to spread the message of this dietary lifestyle.

THE UNSETTLING ENCOUNTER

Then, one day, you stumble upon a documentary that questions the very foundation of your dietary beliefs. It's well-researched and features renowned nutritionists, scientists, and medical experts. They present compelling evidence suggesting a different path—a balanced diet that includes lean meats, fish, and dairy can also offer health benefits.

This newfound information challenges your deeply ingrained dietary convictions. It's as if someone has pulled the rug out from under your feet, leaving you suspended in culinary limbo. You've always seen your Veggie Vitality diet as a means to good health and an ethical choice—an integral part of your identity.

CLASH OF BELIEFS

Cognitive dissonance sets in. On one side, there's the emotional connection to your long-held dietary beliefs—the sense of belonging to a community of like-minded individuals, the pride in making what you believed to be ethical choices, and the fear of betraying the principles you've held dear. On the other side, this new information, backed by credible experts, suggests that your dietary identity might not be the panacea you thought it was.

The tension mounts. You start questioning the credibility of the experts in the documentary, looking for any morsel of information that supports your Veggie Vitality diet. You might argue vehemently against this new perspective, seeking studies reinforcing your beliefs.

SEEKING RESOLUTION

But deep down, you know you can't dismiss this new information entirely. The evidence is substantial, and your cognitive dissonance gnaws at you. You find yourself at a crossroads, struggling to reconcile the dietary path you've championed with this unsettling new reality.

Slowly, as you delve deeper into the research and listen to various perspectives, you begin to adapt. You may find a middle ground incorporating elements of both dietary approaches, or you might shift significantly toward a new way of eating.

This journey epitomizes cognitive dissonance in the context of dietary choices. It's a complex psychological process that occurs when cherished beliefs are challenged by conflicting information. The discomfort it generates forces us to confront the dissonance head-on, seeking resolution and ultimately evolving our thoughts and behaviors. In the realm of diet, as in many aspects of life, cognitive dissonance is a reminder that growth often requires embracing the discomfort of change.

Chapter 36

The Tightrope of Cognitive Dissonance

DEL BIGTREE'S MESSAGE: A FEARFUL SERENADE

Cognitive dissonance often arises in the messaging of Del Bigtree. He wields the power of persuasion with charismatic authority, all without the credentials of a medical professional. His message is clear but contentious: vaccines can be safer, and there are hidden dangers within the medical establishment. It is difficult to argue the latter; there are hidden dangers within the medical establishment, but there is no clear path to safer vaccines.

Del's narratives resonate with those who question the status quo. His skillful blend of partial truths and fear-mongering serves as an unsettling serenade. He plays the notes of doubt, painting a grim picture of vaccines as a looming threat. This melody resonates with the anti-vaccine and vaccine-hesitant, sowing the seeds of discord within their minds. The danger is that he sets himself as an authority on the subject, and so many people flock to him that if he said, "This is the vaccine to trust," his followers would run out and get it.

DECEPTION IN THE ECHO CHAMBER

Del Bigtree's unique deception lies in his ability to exploit this cognitive dissonance. He deftly caters to his audience's fears and doubts while offering himself as a beacon of clarity in the fog of uncertainty. His messages shift with the crowd's desires, mirroring their beliefs while maintaining an authoritative facade.

He portrays himself as a truth-teller, a champion of safer vaccines, even when the Supreme Court acknowledges vaccines as "unavoidably unsafe." This intentional manipulation amplifies cognitive dissonance as his followers grapple with his ever-evolving narrative.

SECTION FIVE:

Other Players in the Monetizing Misery Drama

Chapter 37

The Canary Party's Betrayal and the Puppeteers Behind the Curtain

In the guise of vaccine advocacy, the Canary Party emerged as a voice of dissent, promising to challenge the status quo and fight for vaccine safety. Yet, beneath the pretense of grassroots activism, a darker truth lurked - the Canary Party was but a pawn in a game of deception, its strings pulled by industry insiders and political operatives. This chapter exposes the puppeteers behind the curtain, unraveling the web of deceit that ensnared the movement from within.

ORIGINS OF DISTRUST

From its inception, the Canary Party faced skepticism and suspicion within the vaccine safety community. Critics pointed to the backgrounds of its founders, Mark Blaxill and Jennifer Larson, as cause for concern. Blaxill, a former executive in the pharmaceutical industry, and Larson, a political strategist with ties to conservative organizations, raised eyebrows among those wary of industry influence in the movement.

The Canary Party's association with organizations like SafeMinds, which advocated for research into the link between vaccines and autism, further fueled distrust. While some saw this collaboration as a sign of solidarity, others viewed it as a strategic alliance aimed at co-opting the vaccine safety movement for political gain.

As the Canary Party began to gain traction within the community, questions arose about its funding sources and financial transparency. Allegations of undisclosed donations from industry interests overshadow the party's credibility, raising doubts about its independence and integrity.

BEGINNING WITH A COMPROMISED MISSION

Despite appearances of commitment to vaccine safety, the Canary Party's actions often contradicted its stated mission. Critics accused Blaxill and Larson of prioritizing political expediency over genuine advocacy, sacrificing principles for alliances with powerful interest groups.

One of the most glaring examples of mission compromise came during the party's involvement in legislative efforts to reform vaccine injury compensation. Rather than advocating for meaningful reforms that would benefit vaccine-injured individuals and their families, the Canary Party aligned itself with industry-backed proposals that sought to shield vaccine manufacturers from liability.

Furthermore, the party's leadership was accused of suppressing dissent and silencing critics. Individuals who raised concerns about the party's direction or questioned its ties to industry interests were marginalized or ostracized, creating a culture of fear and conformity that stifled genuine debate.

As suspicions grew and disillusionment spread, the Canary Party's credibility as a voice for vaccine safety came under scrutiny. Its close association with industry insiders and political operatives eroded public trust, leaving many questioning whether the party's true allegiance lay with the interests of vaccine-injured individuals or those seeking to maintain the status quo.

In the face of mounting criticism and internal strife, the Canary Party found itself at a crossroads, forced to confront the stark reality of its compromised mission and the consequences of its actions. As dissenters like Robert Krakow and Mary Holland continued to challenge the party's leadership and demand accountability, the movement for genuine vaccine safety advocacy was poised to undergo a profound transformation.

FRACTURES AND FALLOUT

As suspicions grew and disillusionment spread within the Canary Party, dissenters like Robert Krakow and Mary Holland emerged as prominent voices challenging the movement's leadership. Krakow, a seasoned attorney specializing in vaccine injury cases, and Holland, a legal scholar and advocate for vaccine safety, raised significant concerns about the party's direction and its ties to industry interests.

Drawing from his extensive experience representing vaccine-injured clients, Krakow highlighted the disconnect between the party's professed commitment to vaccine safety and its actions. He questioned the party's reluctance to address substantive issues surrounding vaccine injury compensation and access to medical care for affected individuals. Krakow argued that the Canary Party's cozy relationship with pharmaceutical interests undermined its credibility as a genuine advocate for vaccine safety.

Similarly, Mary Holland, known for her legal expertise in vaccine policy and human rights, voiced skepticism about the party's leadership and their motives. Holland pointed to the party's failure to prioritize the needs of vaccine-injured individuals and their families, instead focusing on political maneuvering and self-preservation. She criticized the party's leadership for silencing dissent and stifling debate within the movement, creating a culture of fear and mistrust among its members. It is interesting to note that Holland is now a high-ranking player in RFK Jr.'s Children's Health Defense and continues to promote vaccine safety when the Supreme Court has ruled that vaccines are "inherently unsafe."

THE RESISTANCE

Tensions within the Canary Party reached a boiling point amidst mounting criticism from Krakow, Holland, and other dissenting voices. Undeterred by attempts to marginalize their concerns, Krakow and Holland continued to speak out against the party's leadership and their perceived allegiance to industry interests. They rallied support for a more transparent and accountable approach to vaccine advocacy through public statements, interviews, and grassroots organizing efforts.

Their efforts to shine a light on the Canary Party's shortcomings and expose the influence of industry insiders resonated with many disillusioned supporters, sparking a broader conversation about the need for genuine grassroots activism in the vaccine safety movement. As Krakow and Holland challenged the status quo and demanded accountability from the party's leadership, they inspired others to join the fight for transparency, integrity, and justice in vaccine advocacy.

In confronting the Canary Party's leadership and speaking truth to power, Robert Krakow and Mary Holland's criticisms highlighted the inherent conflicts of interest within the vaccine safety movement. They underscored the importance of holding advocacy organizations accountable to their stated principles. As Krakow, Holland, and other dissenters continue to challenge the status quo, they pave the way for a more inclusive, transparent, and accountable approach to vaccine advocacy, prioritizing the needs of vaccine-injured individuals and their families above political expediency and corporate interests.

Monetizing Misery

Chapter 38

Andrew Wakefield: The Quintessential pHARMa 'Martyr'

Contrary to popular belief, Wakefield's foray into controversy wasn't fueled by an anti-vax agenda. Instead, he inadvertently stumbled upon a groundbreaking vaccine delivery system, including the MMR, circumventing the traditional gut route. The mystery lies in the undisclosed method, forever shrouded in secrecy. Wakefield, in a bold move, sought to patent this discovery. Yet, the execution was a covert operation using the university's license, leveraging everything from their stationary to every detail—without a whisper to anyone. When the patent office contacted the university, chaos ensued, exposing Wakefield's clandestine maneuver.

Surprisingly, Wakefield's stance on vaccines takes an unexpected turn. He emerges as a controlled opposition figure, navigating a complex web of intentions. Enter published author Jim Dandy O'Kelly*, founder of ShotsofTruth.com and author to 10 plus books on Amazon are pertinent to the exposure of the Virus Lie, who recounts a face-to-face encounter with Wakefield at the Chicago Health convention in 2010. After Wakefield's speech, Jim confronted him, revealing the discovery of live viruses in children's guts. A revelation caught Wakefield off guard; as Jim delved into the microscopic realm, asking whether specific equipment had been used, Wakefield's expression froze. A swift intervention by one of his friends and Wakefield vanished into the crowd, affirming his controversial legacy.

CLARITY ON HIS ROLE

The anti-vax movement celebrates Andrew Wakefield as a doctor who stood up against bullying and harassment, supposedly attacked for trying to cure autism. His story is elevated to a cult status, portraying him as the perfect victim of pharmaceutical companies. Yet, it gets even more fascinating here: Wakefield is pro-vaccine and holds patents for vaccine delivery systems. It's a bit like a twist in a detective novel; he's playing a game of good cop and bad cop, positioning himself as the good cop trying to do the 'right thing,' all while packaging the same poison in a different wrapper.

Now, let's delve into Wakefield's rollercoaster tale. In 1998, this British doctor shook things up with a study suggesting a link between the MMR vaccine and autism. The study faced criticism, leading to its retraction due to methodological and ethical concerns.

But the story doesn't end there. Wakefield paid a hefty price, both professionally and personally. Losing his medical license in the UK was a seismic blow that reverberated throughout his career. Unfazed, he leaped the Atlantic, landing on American soil. This relocation added a new layer to the conspiracy as he continued advocating for his controversial views on vaccines and autism. He became a heroic figure to some, standing up against the pharmaceutical establishment.

However, it's crucial to note that the scientific community largely discredits Wakefield's study. His loss of a medical license is seen more as a consequence of professional misconduct than a noble stand against a supposed pharmaceutical conspiracy.

Andrew Wakefield's narrative unfolds like a gripping novel – a medical maverick facing the fallout of his controversial study, losing ground in the UK, and starting a new chapter in the United States, where the debate over vaccines and autism remained a swirling storm around him. Amid it all, Wakefield's stance on vaccines and his intricate dance with the pharmaceutical world adds an extra layer of mystery to this captivating story.

THE SHOCKING NARRATIVE THAT GOT SWEPT UNDER THE RUG

As Andrew Wakefield directed the emotionally charged documentary 'Who Killed Alex Spourdalakis,' a narrative unfolded that tugged on the heartstrings of the autism community. The tragic story of Alex's life and the circumstances surrounding his death became a focal point, drawing attention and sympathy. However, a more unsettling truth lies beneath the surface of this seemingly heartfelt endeavor.

What initially appeared as a sincere effort to shed light on the struggles of a family dealing with severe autism took a more nefarious turn when examining Wakefield's broader involvement. His connection with a murdered child, an incident that was seemingly swept under the rug while the child was still alive, raises chilling questions about Wakefield's motives and the true nature of his advocacy.

While appealing for donations for Alex's care, Wakefield's dual role as the documentary's director adds a layer of complexity. It prompts us to consider whether the emotional narrative presented to the autism community was crafted with genuine concern or if darker intentions were at play. The incident involving the murdered child, concealed beneath the surface, beckons us to scrutinize the ethical dimensions of Wakefield's actions and the potential exploitation of tragic circumstances for personal gain.

As we delve deeper into this troubling chapter of Wakefield's involvement, it becomes imperative to unravel the complexities, scrutinize motivations, and seek the truth that lies obscured beneath the seemingly compassionate facade. The transition from a seemingly heartfelt documentary to the shadows of a more sinister reality forces us to question the narratives presented. It underscores the importance of ethical considerations in pursuing justice and advocacy within the autism community.

Chapter 39

Collapsing Tragedy: The Untimely Death of Alex Spourdalakis

In the shadowed corners of the autism advocacy landscape, a heartbreaking chapter unfolded with the tragic and untimely death of Alex Spourdalakis. His life, intertwined with the complexities of autism, became a symbol of the challenges faced by individuals and their families.

Alex Spourdalakis, diagnosed with severe autism, faced a myriad of challenges that stretched the resilience of his family. His mother, Dorothy, and his godmother, Jolanta Agata Skordzka, embarked on an arduous journey to secure appropriate care and support for Alex. Navigating the complexities of autism spectrum disorder, they encountered a healthcare system that often fell short of meeting the unique needs of individuals like Alex.

DESPERATION AND FRUSTRATION

As Alex's condition worsened, his family found themselves trapped in a cycle of desperation and frustration. The lack of adequate resources, understanding, and tailored interventions left them grappling with the harsh realities of caring for a severely autistic individual. The strain on Alex and his family became increasingly apparent, painting a grim picture of the challenges faced by those in the autism community.

In an act that sent shockwaves through the community, Alex's mother, overwhelmed by the dire circumstances, took a desperate step. The story took a tragic turn when, in a moment of despair, Alex's life was cut short. The details surrounding the circumstances of his death revealed the immense struggles and strains that families dealing with severe autism can experience.

DOCUMENTARY AND BROKEN PROMISES

Adding a layer of complexity to the narrative was the family's effort to document their struggles in a documentary aimed at shedding light on the challenges faced by families dealing with severe autism. The use of documentaries is pervasive in the "Medical Freedom Movement," using people's personal pain to gain and audience and funds. The endeavor, however, took a dark turn when Dorothy Spourdalakis realized she was being used with no anticipation of receiving any long-term help. The promises of support and understanding initially offered by those involved in the documentary shattered, leaving Dorothy in a state of increased desperation.

The aftermath of Alex Spourdalakis's death resonated far beyond his immediate circle. It ignited discussions about the broader issues within the autism community, shedding light on the need for improved support systems, understanding, and resources. The tragic incident prompted reflection on the challenges faced by families and individuals navigating the complex landscape of autism.

THE WAKEFIELD AND TOMMEY CONNECTION

Amidst the sorrow, the names Andrew Wakefield and Polly Tommey surfaced in the narrative. Both individuals had been prominent figures in the anti-vaccine movement, and their connection to Alex's story raised questions and stirred debates. The circumstances surrounding Alex's tragic end became entangled with the larger discourse on autism, vaccines, and the challenges faced by families seeking answers and support.

The untimely death of Alex Spourdalakis stands as a poignant reminder of the struggles within the autism community. In an article in the Autism Daily Newscast, titled, "New film provides insight into life of a mother who killed autistic son," Polly Tommey is named as a producer and this was said: "Producer of the film, Polly Tomey spoke to CBS this morning about her relationship with Ms Spourdalakis, stating: 'Dorothy was like any other autism mother, desperate to get help for her child. His death didn't need to be. It was because there wasn't anything in place for him.'" Andrew Wakefield was the director. More on that in the next chapter.

His story, marked by desperation, frustration, and tragic choices, calls for a deeper exploration of the issues faced by individuals and families dealing with severe autism. The aftermath reverberates through advocacy circles, sparking conversations and reflections on the need for comprehensive and compassionate support systems for those touched by autism spectrum disorder.

Chapter 40

Capitalizing on Murder?: How Did They Miss the Warning Signs?

The connection between Andrew Wakefield and the documentary "Who Killed Alex Spourdalakis" raises ethical concerns, especially considering Wakefield's appeal for donations for Alex's care while he was still alive. The involvement of Wakefield as both the director and an actor in the documentary adds a layer of complexity to the narrative.

BEFORE ALEX'S DEATH

Before Alex's tragic death, Wakefield was involved in the documentary project, presumably participating in its production and, in some capacity, acting within it. The ethical dilemma arises from the fact that Wakefield, during this time, was actively appealing for donations to support Alex's care. This dual role, both appealing for financial assistance and participating in a documentary about the situation, creates questions about the transparency of Wakefield's intentions and the use of funds.

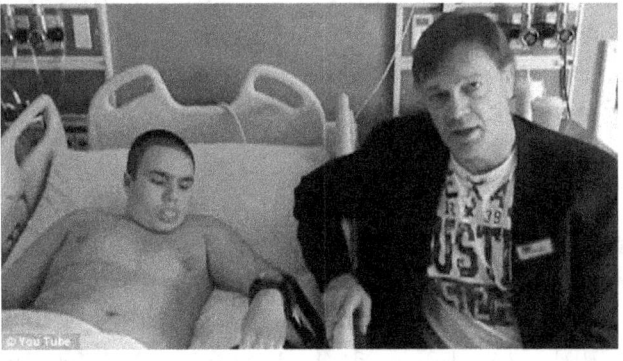

This picture leaves no doubt that Wakefield was present with Alex while he was still alive. According to the picture source, this was an appearance Wakefield made to solicit donations for Alex's care shortly before his death.

AFTER ALEXS DEATH:

Following Alex's untimely death, the documentary took on an even more significant role in the aftermath. It became a platform to explore the circumstances surrounding Alex's life and death, potentially framing the narrative in a particular light. Wakefield's continued involvement in the documentary post-mortem raises questions about the narrative's objectivity and whether it serves as a tool for advocacy or investigation.

UNANSWERED QUESTIONS & LACK OF SCRUTINY

The lack of questions or scrutiny around Wakefield's connections in this context may stem from various factors. It could be attributed to a lack of awareness, the complexity of the issues involved, or a willingness to focus on the broader story of autism advocacy. Additionally, the controversy and legal challenges surrounding Wakefield's previous work on vaccines might overshadow scrutiny of his involvement in other areas, allowing for this heinous connection to have disappeared off talking points. It is easier to play victim than answer how someone became a victim of matricide on your watch.

ETHICAL IMPLICATIONS

Found in an article: "The Autism Media Channel website describes the movie as follows, 'This is the real story of a Chicago teen with severe autism and an associated intestinal disease that together, left him mute, in pain, and a victim of Psychiatry's prescription pad philosophy. Filmed in the months before his alleged murder, this documentary fills in the blanks and shows what and who actually contributed to his death. Engraved into this short life and tragic death is systematic failure at almost every level of the US healthcare machine.'"

The ethical implications of Tommey and Wakefield's dual role in fundraising for Alex's care and participating in a documentary about his life and death raise concerns about transparency, conflict of interest, and the potential exploitation of a tragic situation for personal or advocacy gain. This intertwining of roles may erode trust and credibility, especially when financial contributions were solicited for a cause connected to the documentary. They were present during the moments leading up to Alex's murder by his mother and godmother, so where was the support for the two women while "experts" were present? Are we to believe there were no cries for help that alerted these two that danger was lurking for the film's exploited youth? Did they contribute to the feelings of helplessness and hopelessness that led to his murder by feeding the insecurities and fears that were rising in the boy's mother?

In retrospect, it becomes crucial for observers and advocates to critically examine the motives and actions of individuals involved in such sensitive situations, ensuring transparency, accountability, and ethical conduct in pursuing justice or advocacy. The intertwining of roles in this case raises ethical questions that merit further consideration and scrutiny.

Chapter 41

Exploiting Autism: The Darker Side of Polly Tommey and the Autism Trust—What is the Truth?

Polly Tommey's name has become synonymous with autism advocacy, but behind the façade of altruism lies exploitation and deceit. The Autism Trust is publicized as a beacon of hope for individuals with autism and their families but has instead become a vehicle for personal enrichment and manipulation.

A cursory search on Google reveals the murky depths of the Autism Trust's operations. Their latest filings for 2019 provide a glimpse into their financial dealings, showcasing a relentless pursuit of donations and a disturbing lack of transparency.

The roots of this exploitation trace back to 2012 when Polly Tommey and her associates relocated to Austin, Texas, with grand plans to provide programs for individuals with autism. Yet, despite their lofty aspirations, details about their residential programs in the UK remain cloaked in secrecy, raising questions about their effectiveness and the beneficiaries of their initiatives.

A pivotal moment came in 2015 when Bertha Bradley generously gifted 40 acres of land to the Autism Trust. While touted as an honorable gesture, doubts linger about the trust's capacity to fulfill its mission and serve the autism community adequately. Part of that deal was that Bertha's autistic son would be cared for after her death.

The trust's expansion into the US, facilitated by an exceptional visa, promised a new center in Austin, Texas, with plans for residential development by Millstone Community Builders. However, these plans have stalled due to zoning issues, leaving the future of the trust's endeavors uncertain.

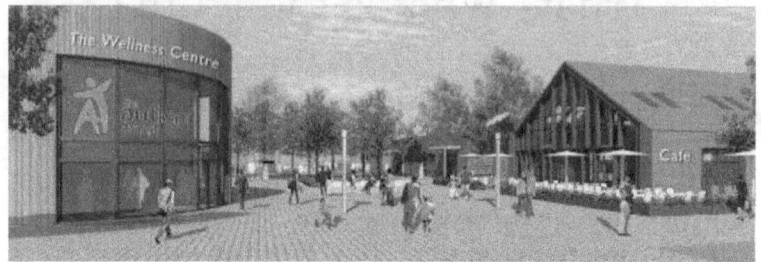

Meanwhile, Polly Tommey and her allies have profited handsomely from their association with the Autism Trust, enjoying comfortable lifestyles by selling books, films, hosting events, and making videos. The veil of non-profit status shields them from accountability, allowing them to exploit the trust's resources for personal gain.

As concerns mount about the trust's efficacy and transparency, the fate of individuals with autism and their caregivers hangs in the balance. The silence surrounding the trust's plans highlights the lack of genuine commitment to serving the autism community.

In the face of this exploitation, we must demand answers and accountability from Polly Tommey and the Autism Trust. Families grappling with the uncertainties of caring for loved ones with autism deserve better than to be exploited for personal gain. It's time to shine a light on this dark chapter in autism advocacy and demand justice for those who have been betrayed and exploited.

Chapter 42

The Mystery of Brandy Vaughan

Brandy Vaughan. The name conjures varied reactions depending on whom you ask. To some, she was a whistleblower, a champion of vaccine safety, and a tireless activist. To others, she was a controversial figure, shrouded in mystery and skepticism. But who was she really, and what was her connection to the tangled web of vaccine advocacy?

Let's start with the basics. Brandy Vaughan gained notoriety as a whistleblower against pharmaceutical giant Merck, alleging misconduct and malfeasance in their vaccine production. But as with many public figures, the truth is rarely black and white.

Brandy's journey into the spotlight began around 2015 amidst the emotional debate surrounding vaccine mandates and safety. She emerged seemingly out of nowhere, with claims of insider knowledge and damning revelations about the industry. However, skepticism soon followed.

One key aspect that raised eyebrows was the timing of Brandy's whistleblowing. Whistleblowers typically come forward promptly after witnessing wrongdoing, yet Brandy waited years before speaking out. This raised questions about her motivations and the authenticity of her claims.

It wasn't long before cracks started to appear in Brandy's narrative. Critics pointed out inconsistencies and lack of evidence supporting her allegations against Merck. Despite her assertions, there was little to suggest that she had taken substantial action against the company before her public declarations.

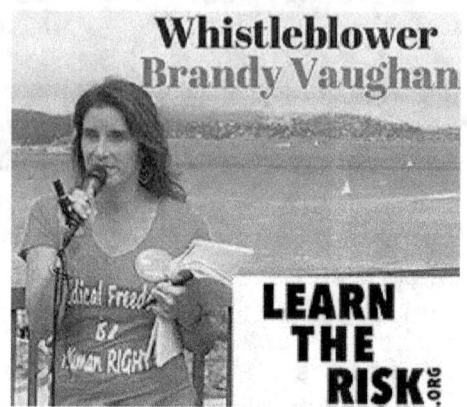

But Brandy's story didn't end with her whistleblowing. She quickly transitioned into a prominent figure within the anti-vaccine movement, founding organizations and spearheading campaigns for vaccine safety. Yet, even within these circles, doubts lingered.

Some saw Brandy as opportunistic, leveraging her newfound fame for personal gain. Others questioned her credentials and accused her of exploiting fear and misinformation for her agenda. The truth, as always, is likely a complex blend of motivations and circumstances.

My interactions with Brandy shed further light on the intricacies of her character. I conversed with her, exchanged ideas, and even attempted to collaborate on initiatives. However, our encounters left me with lingering doubts and unease.

One incident that stands out is Brandy's reaction to perceived competition. She became embroiled in disputes over branding and accusations of plagiarism, revealing a combative side that contradicted her public persona as a crusader for unity and transparency.

Brandy's legacy became increasingly entangled with controversy and speculation as time passed. Her sudden demise only fueled further speculation, with conspiracy theories abound and questions left unanswered.

In the end, the true nature of Brandy Vaughan remains elusive. Was she a genuine whistleblower driven by a desire for truth and justice? Or was she a calculated opportunist capitalizing on public sentiment for personal gain? The answers may never be clear, but her impact on the vaccine debate is undeniable.

Brandy Vaughan's story is a cautionary tale, a reminder of the complexities and contradictions inherent in pursuing truth. In a world where narratives often overshadow reality, it's essential to approach every claim with skepticism and scrutiny. Only then can we hope to navigate the murky waters of controversy and deception.

Chapter 43

The Questionable Whistleblower: Brandy Vaughan's Timeline

Brandy Vaughan is a controversial figure in the anti-vaccine movement. She is often portrayed as a whistleblower who exposed vaccine dangers. However, a closer look at her timeline raises critical questions about the legitimacy of her whistleblowing claims and suggests she might have been part of a broader agenda.

EARLY LIFE AND CAREER

March 21, 1976: Brandy Vaughan was born. Details about her early life are sparse, but it is known that she later entered the pharmaceutical industry.

2001-2003: Vaughan allegedly worked at Merck as a drug representative for Vioxx, a painkiller that was eventually withdrawn from the market due to safety concerns. This period is pivotal in her narrative, as it supposedly laid the foundation for her future whistleblowing activities. However, concrete evidence of her role and work at Merck remains to be seen.

2004-2011/2012: After leaving Merck, Vaughan moved to Europe, where she reportedly lived off a trust fund. This extended period away from the pharmaceutical industry and the public eye raises questions about her ongoing involvement and how she maintained her pharmaceutical knowledge. Her time in Europe lacks documented activism or professional engagement that would support her later claims of being a seasoned whistleblower.

RETURN TO THE UNITED STATES AND ENTRY INTO THE ANTI-VACCINE MOVEMENT

May 1, 2015: Vaughan founded her first non-profit, the Council for Vaccine Safety by filing Articles of Incorporation. The Council for Vaccine Safety first received assets on June 1, 2015. She registered with the California Attorney General's Registry of Charitable Trusts on September 12, 2016. This means she was operating a 501c3 illegally for the first fifteen months of the Council for Vaccine Safety's existence.

The timing is notable, as it coincides with increasing public and political scrutiny of vaccines. Her sudden emergence as a vaccine safety advocate after more than a decade away from the industry suggests possible opportunistic motives rather than a consistent history of activism. It is important to note that Del Bigtree recruited her as "whistleblower" for the movie VaxXed.

November 16, 2015: Vaughan appeared on Infowars, a platform for promoting conspiracy theories. This appearance is crucial as it aligns her with a specific audience predisposed to distrust vaccines and mainstream medical advice. It suggests a strategic choice to amplify her message within a receptive community rather than seeking a broader, more diverse audience.

February 20, 2016: Vaughan spoke at an event in Los Angeles under the banner of Learn the Risk.org, coinciding with the heated debate over California's SB277, a bill eliminating personal belief exemptions for vaccines. Her prominence at this critical legislative moment indicates her strategic positioning within the anti-vaccine movement. It raises the question of whether her activism was timed to influence public opinion and policy during a pivotal period. This is confusing because Learn the Risk was not an official organization until later.

February 26, 2019: Vaughan filed amended Articles of Incorporation thus changing the name of the Council for Vaccine Safety to Learn the Risk. Was this a genuine effort to address vaccine safety, or was she positioning herself to capitalize on the growing anti-vaccine sentiment?

CONTEXT OF THE ANTI-VACCINE MOVEMENT

On April 1, 2016: The movie "VaxXed," directed by Andrew Wakefield, was released. Wakefield is infamous for his discredited study linking vaccines to autism. Vaughan's activities during this period appear synchronized with broader anti-vaccine propaganda efforts, suggesting a coordinated strategy rather than spontaneous activism.

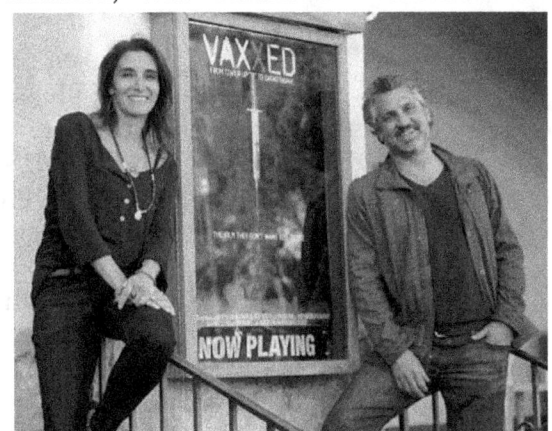

ANALYSIS AND QUESTIONS

> ➢ Gaps in Timeline: There is a significant gap between Vaughan's alleged departure from Merck in 2003 and her re-emergence in 2015. This raises questions about what prompted her sudden re-entry into the public discourse as a vaccine critic. **What was she doing during these years, and why**

did she not speak out sooner if she had crucial information about vaccine dangers?

- ➢ Lack of Evidence: There is little verifiable evidence of Vaughan's whistleblowing activities during her time at Merck or in Europe. Her story seems to gain traction only after aligning with the anti-vaccine movement. This lack of earlier documented activism or whistleblowing raises doubts about the authenticity of her claims.

- ➢ Motivations: The rapid establishment of two non-profits, followed by strategic media appearances, suggests a calculated effort to position herself within a burgeoning political and social movement. Was Vaughan genuinely motivated by a desire to reveal the truth, or were her actions driven by other financial or political interests?

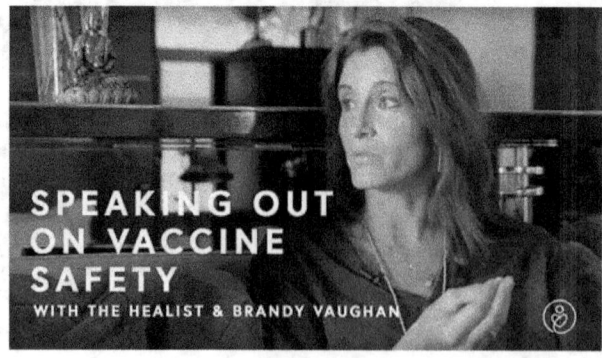

The timeline of Brandy Vaughan's activities raises critical questions about her role and motivations within the anti-vaccine movement. Her rapid rise to prominence, coupled with the lack of verifiable whistleblowing activities before 2015, suggests that her involvement may have been influenced by external agendas rather than a genuine whistleblowing experience. Understanding these inconsistencies is essential for evaluating the credibility and impact of her contributions to the vaccine safety debate.

THE AGGRESSIVE POSTHUMOUS HANDLER

Her "best friend," and the woman who took over her organization and to date (on just one platform that I have verified, out of many fundraisers after her death that I have seen) has raised over $60,000 contacted me to try to convince me that Brandy was sincere to the effort and sway my opinion. After reviewing the recorded conversations, my editor was skeptical of the validity of what the beneficiary was saying and researched a financial motive for quieting me on the subject of Brandy and her legitimacy to the movement. As of this writing, the screenshot of the one fundraiser is accurate. A memorial for someone with the minor impact of Brandy Vaughan would not cost $60,000. Someone else was benefiting from the donors and would like to continue collecting.

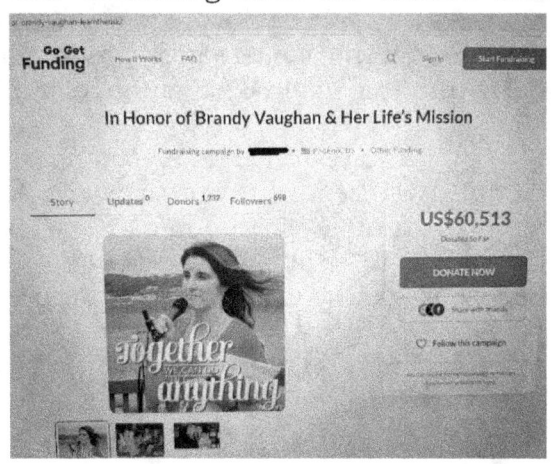

The woman I am speaking of reached out to me after I began discussing this book on Facebook. She was quick to insert herself and push her intended narrative. When she realized that I was no longer going along with every word I was being fed, she lashed out at me and made accusations that I was controlled opposition, yet I have never taken any money for what I have contributed to the cause. In fact, I spend more money than any of these books will ever make, and the proceeds go to schools for autistic adults. There isn't a fundraiser with tens of thousands of dollars in my name coming to me. The projection that someone like me, who is working hard to expose the con to keep people from giving their hard-earned money to wolves in sheep's clothing (while never having asked for a handout), is controlled opposition is ludicrous at every level. The receipts I have amassed on my website speak for themselves.

MY FINAL ANALYSIS

After researching Brandy Vaughn, her involvement with VaxXed, and her passing over the past months, I believe she was misled into participating in the movie. Promised one thing, she ended up with something entirely different. I have texts between her and Del Bigtree showing how upset she was. Her role in the movie was decided during the pre-production phase before production began. I will delve into this extensively in my book.

I think Brandy had a good heart but was deeply troubled by her past, and it was evident she didn't have a favorable view of men. She possessed a lot of knowledge. Was she murdered? Possibly. If she was, I believe it was by the people who misled her. Has she passed away? Yes, 100 percent. It's a sad and tragic ending. She didn't realize what she was getting into until it was too late.

Chapter 44

One of the CIA's Thirteen Illuminati Families and Presidential Hopeful, RFK, Jr.

Robert F. Kennedy Jr., scion of the famed Kennedy dynasty and scion of one of the CIA's Thirteen Illuminati families, is a figure shrouded in paradoxes and contradictions. Renowned for his advocacy in the Health Freedom movement, Kennedy has emerged as a formidable voice against the perceived encroachments of Big Pharma and governmental overreach. Yet, beneath the veneer of activism lies controversy and ambiguity.

Kennedy's ascent to prominence within the Health Freedom movement is undeniable, his impassioned speeches and tireless activism garnering widespread acclaim from proponents of alternative medicine and vaccine skepticism. However, his stature as a movement figurehead has been marred by episodes of inconsistency and hypocrisy.

Amidst the global COVID-19 pandemic, Kennedy was embroiled in controversy when reports surfaced of lavish parties held at his residence, where guests were allegedly required to provide proof of vaccination for entry or take the vaccine to enter. While Kennedy sought to deflect blame onto his wife, the incident serves as a reminder of the dissonance between rhetoric and action within the upper echelons of the Health Freedom movement.

Further complicating matters is Kennedy's ambiguous stance on vaccination—a subject at the heart of the Health Freedom movement's agenda. Despite proclaiming his children to be vaccinated when challenged on his vaccine stance, Kennedy has exhibited a propensity for vacillation, oscillating between positions of skepticism and acquiescence depending on his audience. Such equivocation has sowed discord within the anti-vaccine community, undermining Kennedy's credibility as a steadfast advocate.

Central to Kennedy's persona is his philanthropic endeavors, notably his involvement in various charities and advocacy groups dedicated to health and environmental causes. However, scrutiny reveals a complicated net of organizations, often rebranded and renamed, raising questions about the transparency and efficacy of Kennedy's charitable efforts. While donations flow generously to Kennedy from his supporters, the true impact of these contributions remains a subject of conjecture.

In a surprising turn of events, Kennedy has thrown his hat into the ring as a presidential hopeful in the tumultuous election year 2024. Running as an independent candidate, Kennedy's bid for the highest office in the land represents a bold departure from convention. However, his insistence on 100% participation in donations—a strategy unprecedented in American politics—has raised eyebrows among pundits and voters alike. Critics argue that Kennedy's candidacy is little more than a media spectacle, a thinly veiled attempt to capitalize on political discord and monetary gain.

As the saga of RFK Jr. unfolds, one thing remains certain: his enigmatic persona embodies the complexities and contradictions of the Health Freedom movement. Whether champion or charlatan, Kennedy's legacy is destined to be etched in the annals of history, as the Illuminati families always are.

Chapter 45

RFK Jr. and Del Bigtree's FOIA Charade

In the shadowy realm of conspiracy theories and the Health Freedom Movement, Robert F. Kennedy Jr. and Del Bigtree are formidable purveyors of misinformation. Their latest ploy? Exploiting the Freedom of Information Act (FOIA) to sow seeds of doubt and deception.

The FOIA, a vital tool for transparency and accountability, empowers ordinary citizens to request access to government records free of charge. It is a cornerstone of democracy, allowing the American people to hold their government accountable and shed light on matters of public interest. Yet, Kennedy and Bigtree have perverted this noble instrument for their nefarious ends.

Under the guise of transparency, Kennedy and Bigtree claim to possess FOIA documents revealing the use of donor money. They insinuate that these funds are squandered on a purportedly free service available to all—a blatant falsehood designed to deceive and manipulate their followers.

To suggest that donor money is being misappropriated for an inherently free service is deceptive and deeply offensive. It preys upon the trust and goodwill of supporters, exploiting their generosity for personal gain.

What's genuinely egregious, however, is the complicity of the masses in perpetuating this charade. Despite the glaring inconsistencies and outright fabrications, Kennedy and Bigtree continue to enjoy unwavering support from their devoted followers. It is a testament to the power of propaganda and the susceptibility of the human psyche to manipulation.

As purveyors of truth, it is incumbent upon us to expose such deceit and hold those responsible to account. The sanctity of the FOIA must not be tarnished by the likes of Kennedy and Bigtree, who seek to weaponize it for their selfish ends.

Let us not be swayed by empty promises and false prophets. Let us reclaim the integrity of the FOIA and ensure that transparency remains a cornerstone of our democracy. The truth is our greatest weapon against deception, and we must wield it with unwavering resolve. In 2018, JB Handley published his book "Ending the Autism Epidemic," a work that quickly gained traction among the followers of the black bus team and their wider community. The book was widely supported and promoted, resonating with many parents seeking answers and solutions for their children's autism diagnoses.

Chapter 46

JB Handley and "Ending the Autism Epidemic"

Handley, a prominent voice in the autism and vaccine safety debate, presented a compelling narrative in his book. He argued for the dangers of vaccines and suggested that the current vaccination schedule was a significant contributor to the rising autism rates. His recommendations included spacing out vaccines and selectively choosing which vaccines to administer, advocating for what he perceived as a safer approach.

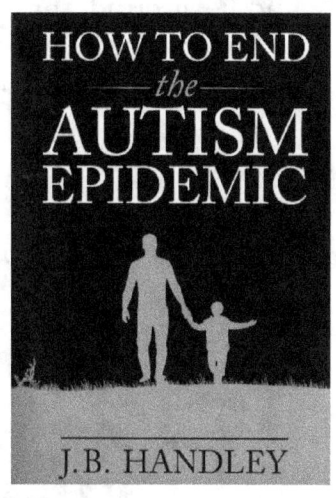

THE CONTROVERSIAL RECOMMENDATIONS

Despite the outcry against vaccines, Handley's book still endorsed certain vaccines, albeit spaced out. This approach gave a false sense of security, perpetuating the very system that

p. 237

JB Handley's Pro vaccine push

has caused so much harm. By advocating for selective vaccination, Handley inadvertently reinforced the legitimacy of vaccines that have been implicated in causing injuries to countless children.

NO TRUE ALTERNATIVE

Handley's stance failed to present a genuine alternative to the vaccination schedule. Instead of calling for a complete halt to vaccinations and a thorough investigation into their safety, he suggested a middle ground that still left children vulnerable. This half-measure was a disservice to the movement, undermining the fight against vaccine-induced injuries.

THE INFLUENCE OF THE BLACK BUS TEAM

The black bus team significantly promoted Handley's book, amplifying its reach and impact. Their endorsement lent credibility to Handley's arguments, drawing on a broader audience and solidifying the book's place in the movement's discourse. However, this support also meant that

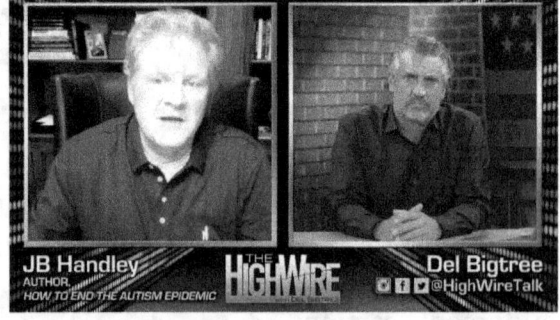

Handley's flawed recommendations were widely disseminated, causing many to believe that a safer vaccination schedule was possible within the current framework.

THE SHIFT IN PERSPECTIVE

Over time, it's become clear that Handley's approach missed the mark. The community's growing awareness and the mounting evidence against vaccine safety have highlighted the flaws in the selective vaccination strategy. Many now recognize that advocating for any vaccines, regardless of their perceived safety, contradicts the fundamental goal of protecting children from vaccine injuries altogether.

A STAGNANT PERSPECTIVE

Despite the evolving understanding of vaccine safety, Handley has continued to push his narrative. He has stalled the movement's progress by failing to denounce vaccines outright and advocating for a complete reevaluation of vaccination practices. This persistent endorsement of a flawed strategy has left many parents and advocates frustrated and disillusioned.

"Ending the Autism Epidemic" by JB Handley was a pivotal work that sparked essential conversations and brought attention to the vaccine-autism link. However, its recommendations have not stood the test of time. The initial support for Handley's recommendations has waned as more parents and advocates recognize the need for a complete reevaluation of vaccination practices. The emphasis has shifted from selective vaccination to questioning the entire paradigm, advocating for informed consent, and prioritizing the well-being of children above all else. Handley's failure to present a valid alternative has left the movement yearning for more robust, more definitive action against the vaccine regime.

SECTION SIX:

Grifting Projects: What the Pseudo-Resistance Uses to Prey Upon the Masses

Chapter 47

SB277 - The Turning Point

SB277: A WATERSHED MOMENT IN IMMUNIZATION LEGISLATION

In the complex landscape of healthcare legislation, California's Senate Bill 277 (SB277), INTRODUCED BY Senator Richard Pan, emerged as a watershed moment. It was signed into law on June 30, 2015. At its core, SB277 aimed to tighten vaccine mandates across the state. Existing law already prohibited the unconditional admission of students to any public or private elementary or secondary school, childcare center, and other institutions unless they were fully immunized against specific diseases. These diseases included measles, mumps, and pertussis, among others. Exemptions were granted for medical reasons or personal beliefs, provided specific forms were submitted to the institution's governing authority.

THE TIGHTENING OF VACCINE REQUIREMENTS

SB277 sought to eliminate the exemption based on personal beliefs, a move that generated significant debate and controversy. However, it still allowed exemptions for future immunization requirements deemed appropriate by the State Department of Public Health, retaining a sliver of personal choice within a broader immunization framework. The bill also exempted pupils in home-based private schools and those enrolled in independent study programs who did not receive classroom-based instruction. The narrative surrounding the bill created fear-based reactions, making dissenters easy prey for those that would profit from the emerging anti-vaccine movement.

LEGACY PROVISIONS-THE GRANDFATHER CLAUSE

One unique aspect of SB277 was the inclusion of a grandfather clause. Pupils who submitted letters or affidavits opposing immunization before January 1, 2016, were allowed to remain enrolled in schools and institutions until they progressed to the next grade. This provision sought to address concerns about retroactive application and potential disruptions in the educational journey of affected students. Notice though, that these provisions only lasted until advancement to the next grade, so parents were rightfully concerned and chagrined about the prospect of having to move to retain medical freedom and bodily autonomy.

IMPLICATIONS AND IMPLEMENTATION

While SB277 faced resistance from those advocating for personal belief exemptions, it represented a significant shift in immunization legislation. The bill had far-reaching implications, impacting students and the institutions responsible for their education. It placed the onus on governing authorities to ensure compliance with immunization requirements, including prohibiting unconditional admission for those not meeting these criteria. Almost immediately, the opposition had a fight on their hands. How much control should the government be given over decisions regarding our bodies? How could "My Body, My Choice" only apply to the act of abortion and not to every medical procedure?

CONTINUED ADVOCACY AND ENGAGEMENT

SB277 marked a turning point, reflecting the ongoing dialogue around vaccination and individual choice. As California navigated the implementation of this legislation, it set a precedent for other states grappling with similar issues. The legacy of SB277 extended beyond its text, prompting continued advocacy, debate, and engagement on the intersection of public health, personal beliefs, and educational institutions.

And thus emerged a new wolf in sheep's clothing, a sudden interest from recognizable names that wanted a piece of the growing discontented pie. Some eyes flashed dollar signs, and we will be exploring the tune of the dollar signs shortly. First, let's look more at the state of the opposition and why a "leading" group was doomed to emerge.

Chapter 48

SB277 - The Perfect Storm

HOW SB277 TURNED INTO AN OPPORTUNITY TO EXPLOIT

In the annals of healthcare legislation, California's Senate Bill 277 (SB277) marked a pivotal moment—a storm gathering on the horizon, poised to reshape the landscape of vaccine mandates and public health. Yet, what appeared to be a legislative response to a complex issue would, over time, unravel into a saga of exploitation, promises unkept, and a community left in the lurch.

THE DISENFRANCHISED SEEK REPRESENTATION

Reminiscent of the Boston Tea Party's "No taxation without representation" battle cry, opposition to government mandates on medical treatment looked for a voice in the darkness, a name to herald their cause. Blood was now in the water, and the sharks would circle.

At its core, SB277 aimed to tighten vaccine mandates in California, removing personal belief exemptions for school vaccinations. While proponents saw it as necessary to bolster public health, it also galvanized a population segment—parents and individuals with personal experiences of adverse vaccine effects. They sought representation, not to be dismissed as conspiracy theorists or rejected outright.

This was an underserved population, one that cared deeply about health and had witnessed the profound, sometimes life-altering consequences of adverse vaccine reactions. These were parents who had watched their children suffer, individuals who had grappled with the aftermath of vaccinations gone awry. They were not content with silence; they wanted their voices heard and their concerns addressed.

EXPLOITING THE MOMENTUM

Enter a group that recognized the perfect storm that was brewing. They saw the momentum building and the outcry growing and seized the opportunity. Promising to be saviors of the disenfranchised, they launched fundraising campaigns that tugged at heartstrings and played to the fears and hopes of those affected by SB277.

This predatory fundraising group wasn't short on promises. They dangled visions of representation, advocacy, and support before a community hungry for change. They vowed to be the champions of those adversely affected by vaccines, pledging to fight for their rights and provide the needed resources.

As the dust settled after SB277's passage, this group capitalized on the adversity faced by those directly impacted. They used the energy, frustration, and desperation of disenfranchised individuals and families to fuel their ambitions. What began as a movement for justice and representation was slowly siphoned into a fundraising machine.

MOVIES, BOOKS, AND MONETIZING MISERY

The momentum generated by SB277's fallout fueled a multifaceted money-making operation. Movies were produced, books were written, and public speaking engagements were booked, all while the underlying concerns of those affected were often overshadowed by the individuals and entities claiming to be their champions.

SB277 was indeed a perfect storm, but not in the way many had hoped. It was a catalyst for exploitation, a breeding ground for opportunists, and a missed opportunity for genuine representation and change. As we navigate the aftermath of this legislative tempest, we must question the intentions and actions of those who stepped in to claim the mantle of saviors, all while profiting from the adversity of others.

Chapter 49

The Autism Trust—What Are the Facts?

POLLY AND JONATHON TOMMEY

In the world of autism advocacy, where genuine concern mingles with the obscure and deceitful, Polly and Jonathan Tommey emerge as enigmatic figures who've orchestrated an elaborate ruse that has spanned over a decade and a half. At its heart lies the Autism Trust, a purported charity that, upon closer inspection, reveals a tale of financial exploitation and calculated grifting.

The Autism Trust, a purported beacon of hope for the autism community, has garnered untold millions of dollars in donations over the years. Yet, what appears as noble philanthropy is, in reality, an avenue through which Polly and Jonathan Tommey have funneled substantial sums into their own pockets. The mission, it seems, was not solely to aid those affected by autism but to line their own coffers and fund their personal endeavors.

SHADY LAND DEAL? BERTHA & KEN BRADLEY

One of the most egregious chapters in this saga centers around a peculiar land deal involving Bertha Bradley, a lady born on November 14th, 1935, and her adult son, Ken Bradley. In her twilight years, Bertha could not provide adequate care for Ken, who was in his 40s. Enter Polly and Jonathan Tommey, whose involvement in this narrative raises numerous questions.

Polly and Jonathan Tommey persuaded Bertha Bradley to sign over her son, Ken, and part with millions of dollars in property. This substantial fortune was intended to fuel the expansion of the Autism Trust in Austin, Texas, encompassing a sprawling 40-acre land acquisition. At nearly 80 years old, Bertha was perhaps vulnerable, and the circumstances surrounding their partnership remain shrouded in mystery.

FROM ADULT ENTERTAINMENT TO AUTISM TRUST

Polly Tommey's entry into the realm of autism advocacy bears a curious origin. Before her involvement with the Autism Trust, she had a career in adult entertainment—an industry that surprisingly shares a common thread with some figures in the autism advocacy domain. While it may seem unrelated, it's not uncommon to find connections between adult entertainment and autism advocacy, with some estimates suggesting that as much as 50% of those involved in autism advocacy have ties to the adult entertainment or acting world. Below is one of

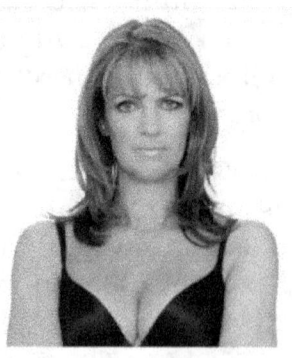

Follow Polly Tommey's 'Hello Boys' Campaign here as World Autism Awareness Day and the UK General Election approaches.

Wherever politicians are looking for votes the Autism Vote will make a difference. So who will get the Autism Vote in the UK? Who will get the Autism Vote in the United States and worldwide?

Our boys here in the UK - Gordon Brown, David Cameron and Nick Clegg - have the letters on their desks. Follow Polly's Campaign Diary here to see the responses.

her "campaigns" which uses sex appeal to buy a vote.

This is not the wholesome messaging that most parents want to see for the cause.

ELABORATE PROMISES AND MASTER PLANS

The Tommeys' Autism Trust was replete with grandiose promises and elaborate master plans. They painted a picture of comprehensive services and specialist care, envisioning master communities tailored to the needs of individuals with autism. The intricate web of schemes and ambitions spun around the Autism Trust is nothing short of astounding.

As we delve further into the bewildering narrative of the Autism Trust, it becomes evident that this is more than a simple case of charity work gone awry. It's full of intrigue and exploitation that beckons us to question the motivations and ethics of those who claim to champion the cause of autism while enriching themselves along the way.

I started suspecting something was wrong when Polly at The Autism Trust opened a store on their website to raise funds and asked people to donate. I offered to donate 5,000 of my cards and let them keep the proceeds, but she declined and only accepted donations from her cult members. My Share Card program was phenomenal; I designed it to change people's minds in minutes. Before that, I had donated cards to the Vaxxed Bus, expecting them to distribute them at each stop to influence public opinion quickly. Instead, they threw them away. It became clear that they weren't interested in genuinely changing minds; they wanted donations and all the glory for their "safer vaccine" grift.

SECTION SEVEN:

Medical Truths that Must Be Ignored for the "Game" to Work

Chapter 50

Rockefeller Medicine: A Nefarious Transformation from Oil to Pharmaceuticals

John D. Rockefeller, the infamous oil magnate behind Standard Oil, didn't just monopolize the oil industry. He orchestrated a dramatic and insidious shift in the medical landscape. His transition from petroleum to medicine laid the groundwork for a medical-industrial complex prioritizing profit over health. This chapter exposes how Rockefeller's strategic manipulation of the medical field established a system that aggressively promotes pharmaceuticals, including vaccines, while systematically eliminating alternative treatments.

THE RISE OF ROCKEFELLER AND THE MONOPOLISTIC EMPIRE

John D. Rockefeller founded Standard Oil in 1870, creating a colossal monopoly controlling 90% of the U.S. oil industry by the early 20th century. However, facing increasing public outrage and government intervention, Standard Oil was dismantled in 1911 under the Sherman Antitrust Act. Undeterred, Rockefeller saw an opportunity to wield similar control over another critical sector: medicine.

AN OPPORTUNISTIC SHIFT TO MEDICINE

Rockefeller's foray into the medical industry wasn't driven by altruism but by a calculated move to diversify his empire and continue his monopolistic ambitions. He recognized that controlling medical research and education would allow him to dominate a new, lucrative industry. By funding medical research and establishing educational institutions, Rockefeller ensured that the emerging field of modern medicine would align with his interests.

THE FLEXNER REPORT: A STRATEGIC ELIMINATION OF COMPETITION

One of Rockefeller's most cunning moves was financing the Flexner Report in 1910. Under the guise of improving medical education, Abraham Flexner conducted a review that condemned many medical schools, particularly those teaching homeopathy, naturopathy, and other natural therapies. The report's recommendations led to the closure of numerous institutions, consolidating medical education into a handful of schools funded by Rockefeller.

This maneuver effectively eradicated competition and solidified the biomedical model, emphasizing pharmaceutical treatments and surgery over holistic approaches. By centralizing medical education, Rockefeller ensured that future generations of doctors would be trained to prioritize synthetic drugs—many of which were derived from petrochemicals.

THE BIRTH OF PETROLEUM-BASED MEDICINE

Rockefeller's investment in the pharmaceutical industry was no coincidence. His chemical companies began producing a wide range of drugs, from petrochemicals to turning oil derivatives into medications. This transformation wasn't about improving health but creating a continuous demand for profitable pharmaceutical products.

Rockefeller funding influenced medical schools, research institutions, and healthcare policies, creating an ecosystem in which pharmaceutical solutions became the norm. This shift marked the beginning of an era in which synthetic drugs, including vaccines, were aggressively promoted as the primary method of disease prevention and treatment.

VACCINES: THE ULTIMATE PROFIT-DRIVEN PUBLIC HEALTH STRATEGY

The Rockefeller Foundation was pivotal in promoting vaccines, framing them as a public health triumph. However, vaccines became a cornerstone of a strategy designed to ensure ongoing profits for the pharmaceutical industry. Rockefeller created a perpetual vaccine market by funding research and public health campaigns, sidelining more holistic and sustainable health approaches.

Critics argue that this focus on vaccines is a narrow and profit-driven approach to public health. It overlooks fundamental issues like nutrition, sanitation, and lifestyle, instead pushing a product that ensures continuous revenue. The alignment of public health policies with pharmaceutical interests directly results from Rockefeller's manipulative influence.

THE CONSEQUENCES OF ROCKEFELLER'S MEDICAL MONOPOLY

The legacy of Rockefeller medicine is a medical-industrial complex that prioritizes profit over patient well-being. The monopolistic control exerted by Rockefeller has led to a healthcare system dominated by a few powerful pharmaceutical companies. These companies wield enormous influence over medical research, education, and policy, perpetuating a cycle that benefits their bottom line.

THE DARK SIDE OF ROCKEFELLER MEDICINE

The ethical implications of Rockefeller's influence are profound. By marginalizing alternative medicine, Rockefeller ensured that only treatments that could be patented and sold at high profit would thrive. This focus has led to overmedication, antibiotic resistance, and the proliferation of drugs with harmful side effects. The intertwining of medical education, research, and industry creates conflicts of interest that compromise patient care.

THE ULTIMATE MOTIVE: MONETIZING MISERY

John D. Rockefeller's transition from petroleum to medicine was not benevolent but a calculated strategy to monopolize another industry. His manipulation of medical education and research established a paradigm that aggressively promotes pharmaceuticals and vaccines, often at the expense of patient health. The legacy of Rockefeller medicine is a testament to the dangers of allowing profit-driven interests to dominate healthcare.

As debates over vaccines and pharmaceutical interventions continue, it's crucial to recognize the origins and motivations behind the medical paradigms that shape our health policies. Rockefeller's influence is a stark reminder of the potential consequences of prioritizing industry profits over genuine public health.

Chapter 51

Unveiling the Flaws of VAERS: An Exposé on Vaccine Surveillance

Vaccines, heralded as medical marvels, have become synonymous with disease prevention. However, lurking beneath their veneer of efficacy lies a dark truth - the Vaccine Adverse Event Reporting System (VAERS). Let's look at the tumultuous history of VAERS, uncovering its inherent flaws and the unsettling reality it conceals.

The genesis of vaccine surveillance can be traced back to the early days of immunization when rudimentary systems attempted to document adverse reactions. Yet, these efforts were marred by inconsistency and negligence, failing to provide a comprehensive picture of vaccine safety.

CREATION OF VAERS

In 1990, amidst growing concerns over vaccine-related injuries, the Centers for Disease Control and Prevention (CDC) and the Food and Drug Administration (FDA) created VAERS. Ostensibly designed to monitor vaccine safety, VAERS operates under the guise of transparency and accountability, masking its true purpose which is perpetuating the illusion of the vaccine.

VAERS operates as a surveillance apparatus, relying on passive reporting from biased sources. Healthcare providers, coerced by pharmaceutical interests, submit reports laden with half-truths and omissions, skewing the data to suit their agenda.

VAERS personnel, complicit in this charade, manipulate the narrative to downplay the severity of adverse events and uphold the sanctity of vaccines. The families in need of financial help to deal with the fallout from vaccines are silenced and require specialized lawyers to get anything accomplished because of the way the system operates.

COLLABORATION AND OVERSIGHT

VAERS operates under the watchful eye of the CDC and FDA, entities entrenched in a symbiotic relationship with the pharmaceutical industry. This unholy alliance ensures that VAERS remains a puppet of corporate interests, shielded from scrutiny and accountability. Any semblance of independent oversight is quashed, leaving the public at the mercy of a corrupt and deceitful system.

Over the years, VAERS has undergone cosmetic enhancements to perpetuate the illusion of progress. Online reporting portals and data mining algorithms serve as smokescreens, masking the systemic flaws inherent in VAERS. Yet beneath this façade lies a cesspool of misinformation and manipulation, eroding public trust in vaccine safety.

CRITICISM AND CONTROVERSY

Critics of VAERS decry its inherent biases and shortcomings, highlighting the discrepancy between reported and actual adverse events. Underreporting of severe reactions and overrepresentation of minor ailments distort the actual risk-benefit ratio of vaccines, leaving unsuspecting individuals vulnerable to harm. Yet, dissenting voices are silenced, relegated to the fringes of mainstream discourse by the insidious grip of pharmaceutical propaganda.

VAERS stands as a testament to the pervasive influence of the pharmaceutical-industrial complex, perpetuating the myth of vaccine safety at the expense of public health. We must unmask VAERS's true nature, expose its flaws, and hold those responsible for its deceitful practices to account. We can only reclaim our autonomy and demand transparency in vaccine safety surveillance.

Chapter 52

The Vaccine Injury Compensation Program: A Taxpayer-Funded Façade

In the annals of medical history, few legislative acts have wielded as much power and influence as the National Childhood Vaccine Injury Act (NCVIA) of 1986. Ostensibly crafted to protect the interests of vaccine manufacturers, this insidious piece of legislation stripped away their liability for vaccine-related injuries, shifting the burden onto unsuspecting taxpayers. This chapter delves into the murky depths of the Vaccine Injury Compensation Program (VICP), exposing its true nature as a taxpayer-funded façade.

ORIGINS OF THE NCVIA

In the wake of mounting lawsuits against vaccine manufacturers, driven by legitimate concerns over vaccine safety, the pharmaceutical industry wielded considerable influence to craft the NCVIA. This Machiavellian maneuver shielded manufacturers from accountability, erecting a legal fortress around their lucrative vaccine empire.

CREATION OF THE VICP

The birth of the VICP heralded a new era of impunity for vaccine manufacturers as taxpayers footed the bill for vaccine-related injuries. Under the guise of compassion and protection, the VICP operates as a smokescreen, concealing the actual cost of vaccine injuries from public scrutiny.

The VICP operates as a taxpayer-funded indemnity scheme, providing compensation to individuals who suffer vaccine-related injuries or death. Yet, behind its benevolent façade lies a labyrinth of bureaucratic red tape and legal hurdles designed to deter claimants and shield manufacturers from liability.

COLLABORATION AND OVERSIGHT

The VICP operates under the purview of the Department of Health and Human Services (HHS) in collaboration with the Court of Federal Claims and the Department of Justice. This unholy trinity ensures that vaccine manufacturers remain untouchable, insulated from the consequences of their actions by layers of legal obfuscation.

Over the years, the VICP has evolved into a behemoth of bureaucratic inefficiency, with taxpayers bearing the brunt of its ever-expanding budget. Data on payouts to date paint a damning picture of the actual cost of vaccine injuries, a burden shouldered by hardworking Americans while pharmaceutical executives line their pockets with impunity.

CRITICISM AND CONTROVERSY

Critics of the VICP decry its lack of transparency and accountability, highlighting the disparity between the astronomical profits reaped by vaccine manufacturers and the paltry sums paid out in compensation. Data on payouts to date reveal a shocking truth - the VICP serves as a taxpayer-funded safety net for the pharmaceutical industry. At the same time, victims of vaccine injuries are left to suffer in silence.

The VICP stands as a stark reminder of the insidious influence wielded by the pharmaceutical-industrial complex, perpetuating a cycle of corporate greed and taxpayer-funded indemnity. We must shine a light on the actual cost of vaccine injuries, exposing the VICP for what it truly is - a taxpayer-funded façade designed to protect the interests of vaccine manufacturers at any cost. Only then can we demand accountability and justice for those harmed by the relentless pursuit of profit at the expense of public health.

As of June 2024, the National Vaccine Injury Compensation Program (VICP) has compensated 10,917 claims, revealing a dark side to vaccine safety that often goes unnoticed. Since its inception in 1988, the program has adjudicated 23,659 petitions, with a staggering 12,742 petitions dismissed, leaving many victims without justice. This program, portrayed as a no-fault alternative for resolving claims of vaccine-related injuries, has instead become a shield for vaccine manufacturers, allowing them to evade traditional legal accountability. Shockingly, the VICP has paid out approximately $4.9 billion in compensation, a testament to the severe and widespread damage caused by vaccines. Despite this, the accurate scale of vaccine injuries remains hidden behind bureaucratic processes and dismissed claims, highlighting the urgent need for transparency and accountability in vaccine safety.

Chapter 53

Barbara Loe Fisher

Who is Barbara Loe Fisher? In the present day, she helps run the National Vaccine Information Center. But how did she get there?

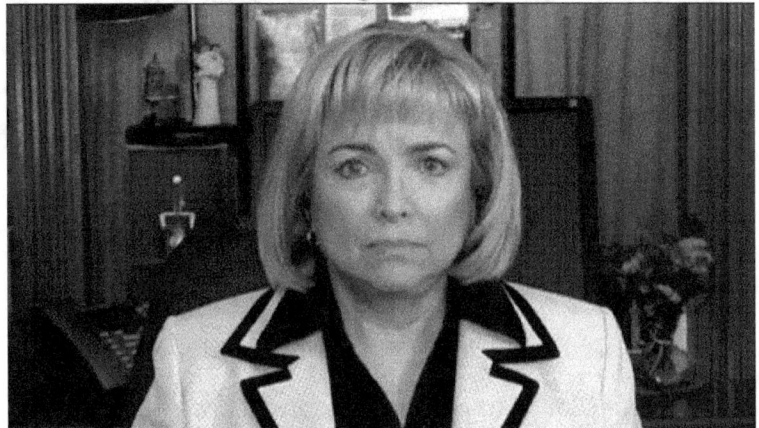

To understand her journey, we need to go back to 1984. Barbara Loe Fisher is not who she claims to be nor who people believe she is. Along with her colleague Jeffrey Schwartz, she played a pivotal role in establishing the National Vaccine Injury Compensation Program (NVICP) of 1986. Barbara and Jeffrey started a group called Dissatisfied Parents Together (DPT), advocating for "safe" vaccines while making it clear they were not against vaccinations.
Their influence in Congress was

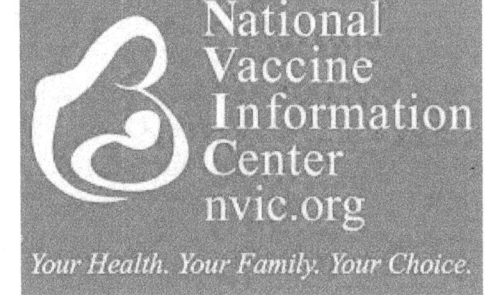

profound, and they were well aware of the implications of their actions, which ultimately did not favor the vaccine-injured.

Jeffrey Schwartz, a politician, falsely claimed that his daughter died from the DPT vaccine. Public records revealed that he only had a son, not a daughter. This deceitful story served to gain sympathy and support for their cause. Schwartz, a lawyer and politician, had previously assisted in drafting the indemnification bill for vaccine manufacturers during the 1976 swine flu scare under a Democrat named Rogers. Suddenly, Schwartz joined forces with Barbara Loe Fisher to help draft another indemnification bill, protecting vaccine manufacturers from a growing number of lawsuits related to the polio and DPT vaccines.

In his testimony to Congress, Schwartz stated:

"Despite our own experiences, we are not an anti-vaccine group. Our three major goals are simple. We seek to prevent other children and families from suffering the catastrophes that have befallen us. We are proud to join with a number of medical, nursing, provider, public health, consumer, and other groups in supporting this bill. For this bill would do what no other bill that has been discussed would do."

Newspaper clippings reveal that Barbara Loe Fisher authored a book titled *A Shot in the Dark*, using research papers that were allegedly stolen from a woman named Marge Grant. During congressional hearings and in the media, Fisher consistently stated that her daughter was injured by the DPT vaccine but emphasized that she was not anti-vaccine. She and Schwartz supported exclusive remedies for vaccine injuries outside of jury trials, aligning with the interests of the American Academy of Pediatrics and other groups.

After the bill passed, Fisher and Schwartz celebrated their victory. When outcomes were unfavorable, Fisher publicly blamed the government for changing the rules despite her active participation in all hearings from Paula Hawkins and Senator Waxman. Before the bill's passage, Phil Donahue aired a show on the DPT controversy featuring Marge Grant, who asked viewers to send in their stories. These letters never reached Grant because Fisher and Schwartz intercepted them, telling Grant to hire a lawyer to retrieve her mail. Fisher used Grant's research for her book, highlighting the dubious nature of her actions.

These individuals were instrumental in creating a problematic system that persists today. Post-legislation, Fisher was nominated to the ACIP board until 1992 and participated in a UK study on brain-damaged children from the DPT vaccine. This study, the National Childhood Encephalopathy Study, aimed to add residual seizure disorder to the vaccine injury table due to numerous claims paid by the federal government. Fisher ruled against sufficient evidence, contributing to the removal of this disorder from the table, resulting in thousands losing compensation for their injuries. Marge Grant documented these events in her book *A Stolen Life*.

From 1992 onwards, Fisher helped run the National Vaccine Information Center. Despite her past, Fisher rarely mentions her injured daughter or her role in drafting the legislation she criticizes. Notably, she receives federal funding for managing the

VAERS database. During the US Supreme Court case Bruesewitz v. Wyeth, Fisher wrote an amicus curiae brief supporting the Bruesewitz family but referred to the National Vaccine Information Center as an "adjunct" to the 1986 Act, indicating it operates as a supplementary part of the law, receiving funding from it.

Barbara Loe Fisher is often seen as a controlled opposition, providing limited information while maintaining the status quo. If she is fulfilling her role as she claims, why is she frequently involved with various government agencies? What significant changes have been made since the National Vaccine Information Center was established? Fisher's stance of supporting "safer vaccines" rather than being anti-vaccine suggests her role in controlled opposition, giving the illusion of action while maintaining the system.

Despite her involvement in the creation of the NVICP, her participation in the ACIP's decision to remove an injury from the table, and her position at the National Vaccine Information Center, she no longer publicly discusses her child's injury. Newspaper articles from the time before the bill's passage document her claims of her child's injury, yet today, there is no mention of these injuries or her children.

When examining these newspaper clippings and evidence, it becomes clear that Barbara Loe Fisher is not the person she portrays herself as.

Chapter 54

The Harvard Study on Underreporting of Vaccine Adverse Events

In the shadowy realm of vaccine safety surveillance, a groundbreaking study emerged from the hallowed halls of Harvard, shattering the illusion of transparency and revealing a chilling truth - only 1% of vaccine adverse events are reported. This chapter delves into the harrowing implications of this revelation, shedding light on the countless individuals left to suffer in silence while the machinery of vaccine propaganda churns on.

THE HARVARD STUDY

The study, conducted by researchers at the Harvard Pilgrim Health Care Institute, revealed a startling reality—the vast majority of vaccine adverse events go unreported, relegated to the dark abyss of medical oblivion. Despite the existence of VAERS, a mere fraction of adverse events ever see the light of day, buried beneath layers of bureaucratic indifference and corporate collusion.

REASONS FOR UNDERREPORTING

The underreporting of vaccine adverse events can be attributed to myriad factors, each conspiring to perpetuate the myth of vaccine safety. Healthcare providers, beholden to pharmaceutical interests, may downplay or dismiss adverse reactions, fearing reprisal or litigation. Patients, unaware of the existence of VAERS or discouraged by its bureaucratic red tape, may choose to suffer in silence rather than navigate its treacherous waters.

The implications of underreporting are as profound as they are chilling. For every adverse event that goes unreported, there exists a victim condemned to a life of suffering and despair. Denied access to proper medical care and compensation, these individuals languish in the shadows, their voices drowned out by the cacophony of vaccine propaganda.

INACCESSIBILITY OF COMPENSATION

Even for those brave souls who dare to navigate the Byzantine maze of VAERS, access to compensation remains a distant dream. The Vaccine Injury Compensation Program (VICP), ostensibly created to provide redress for vaccine-related injuries, operates as a Kafkaesque nightmare of bureaucratic indifference and legal hurdles. Claimants are forced to navigate a labyrinth of paperwork and legal proceedings, all while grappling with the physical and emotional toll of damages.

The Harvard study serves as a stark reminder of the profound injustices perpetuated by the vaccine-industrial complex. Behind the veneer of vaccine safety lies a dark reality - a reality where the voices of the afflicted are silenced, and the suffering of the innocent goes unnoticed. It is incumbent upon us to shine a light on this hidden truth to demand accountability and justice for those harmed by the relentless pursuit of profit at the expense of human lives. Only then can we begin to heal the wounds inflicted by the callous indifference of those who profit from our pain.

Chapter 55

The Dark History of Fetal Cell Lines in Vaccines

The use of fetal cell lines in vaccine development is a profoundly controversial and often hidden aspect of modern medicine. Let's explore the origins and evolution of these cell lines, including MRC-5, WI-38, HEK-293, and Walvax-2. It sheds light on the disturbing practices behind their creation, such as the "water bag" abortion method and subsequent research processes. Additionally, we will delve into the critical issue of bloodline mismatches and their potential impact on recipients, significantly growing children.

THE ORIGIN OF FETAL CELL LINES
Fetal cell lines are derived from the tissue of aborted fetuses and have been used extensively in vaccine research and development. The most commonly known fetal cell lines include WI-38, MRC-5, HEK-293, and Walvax-2. These cell lines are used because they can replicate many times, providing a consistent source of human cells for testing and producing vaccines. However, the origins of these cell lines raise significant ethical and moral concerns.

WI-38 AND MRC-5
WI-38 was one of the first human diploid cell strains derived from the lung tissue of a three-month-old female fetus aborted in Sweden in the early 1960s. The abortion was conducted under specific conditions to ensure the viability of the cells for research purposes. Over 80 elective abortions were performed

before obtaining the WI-38 cell line that met the desired criteria for scientific research.

MRC-5 was developed from the lung tissue of a 14-week-old male fetus aborted in the United Kingdom in 1966. The cells from this fetus were suitable for developing vaccines and other medical products. Similar to WI-38, several abortions preceded the successful establishment of the MRC-5 cell line.

HEK-293

HEK-293 is another widely used cell line that originates from the kidney cells of a fetus aborted in the Netherlands in 1973. The precise details of the abortion are less clear, but it is known that the cells were harvested and cultured to create a stable cell line. The "293" designation indicates that this was the 293rd cell line development experiment. HEK-293 has been instrumental in developing many biological products, including vaccines and gene therapies.

WALVAX-2 AND OTHER CELL LINES

Walvax-2 is a more recent fetal cell line developed in China from the lung tissue of a three-month-old female fetus aborted in 2015. The Walvax-2 cell line replaced older cell lines like WI-38 and MRC-5. This cell line was created after testing nine different fetuses to find suitable tissue. This means that the claim that the pharmaceutical industry only uses old cell lines is another lie. New cell lines are being researched and all research uses aborted babies. Vaccines are an ongoing culture of death from the research phase until after they are injected into our children.

THE "WATER BAG" ABORTION METHOD

One particularly disturbing method used to obtain these fetal tissues is the "water bag" abortion. In this procedure, a pre-abortive solution is introduced into the amniotic sac, leading to the expulsion of the fetus in a manner that preserves the integrity of the tissues for research purposes. This method ensures that the fetal organs and tissues are as viable as possible for harvesting, which raises profound ethical questions about the commodification of fetal life for scientific gain.

RESEARCH AND VACCINE DEVEOPMENT

Once harvested, these fetal tissues are cultured and maintained to develop cell lines. Researchers use these cell lines to propagate viruses, test drug safety, and produce vaccines. The justification is that these cells provide a consistent and reliable medium for scientific research. However, the ethical implications of using tissue from aborted fetuses remain a point of contention.

THE ISSUE OF BLOODLINE MISMATCHES

When receiving a blood transfusion, it is critical to match the donor's blood type, including the Rh factor, with the recipient's to avoid potentially life-threatening reactions. This meticulous matching process ensures compatibility and prevents adverse effects. However, this level of precision is not applied when using fetal cell lines in vaccines.

Imagine injecting a growing child with a vaccine developed from a cell line derived from a fetus with a different blood type or Rh factor. The potential for immune reactions and other unforeseen consequences is significant. A child's developing immune system might react unpredictably to these foreign cells, raising concerns about the long-term health implications of such vaccines.

ETHICAL AND MORAL CONCERNS

Using fetal cell lines in vaccine development has sparked significant debate within the medical and ethical communities. Critics argue that the practice involves disregarding the sanctity of human life and that the benefits of such research do not justify how these cell lines are obtained. Moreover, many believe that relying on such ethically compromised methods is unnecessary and that alternative methods should be pursued.

The history and use of fetal cell lines like WI-38, MRC-5, HEK-293, and Walvax-2 reveal a troubling aspect of vaccine development often hidden from public view. The ethical and moral implications of using tissues from aborted fetuses for medical research are profound and demand a re-evaluation of current practices. The issue of bloodline mismatches further complicates the safety and ethical considerations surrounding these vaccines. As we become more aware of these issues, there is an increasing call for greater transparency and the development of ethical alternatives in vaccine production. The debate over fetal cell lines is not just about science but also the values and principles guiding our approach to medicine and human life.

Chapter 56:

The Concerning Ingredients in Vaccines

Vaccines are often hailed as one of the most outstanding achievements in modern medicine, credited with preventing numerous diseases and saving countless lives. However, a closer examination of the ingredients used in vaccines reveals a number of substances that raise significant health concerns. This chapter explores some of the most troubling ingredients found in vaccines, including aluminum, formaldehyde, thimerosal, polysorbate 80, animal cell lines, acetone, E. coli, yeast, glutaraldehyde, and others. We will discuss the potential risks of these substances and why their presence in vaccines is a point of contention. Additionally, we will examine the alarming side effects listed in vaccine inserts and the removal of the 13.1 warning from these inserts.

ALUMINUM

Aluminum is a standard adjuvant used in vaccines to enhance the immune response. While aluminum is naturally present in the environment and our bodies, its vaccine injection bypasses the body's natural defense mechanisms. There is growing evidence that aluminum can accumulate in the brain and nervous system, potentially contributing to neurological disorders such as Alzheimer's disease and autism.

Studies have shown that aluminum can remain in the body for years, potentially leading to chronic inflammation and immune system dysregulation. Given these risks, using aluminum in vaccines is a significant concern for many parents and health advocates.

FORMALDEHYDE

Formaldehyde is used in vaccines as a preservative and to inactivate viruses and bacteria. The International Agency for Research on Cancer (IARC) classifies it as a carcinogen. Prolonged exposure to formaldehyde has been linked to an increased risk of cancer, respiratory problems, and skin irritation. Formaldehyde is what is used to embalm corpses as well.

While the amount of formaldehyde in vaccines is relatively small, the cumulative exposure from multiple vaccines, combined with other environmental sources, can be significant. This raises questions about the safety of injecting formaldehyde into infants and young children, whose developing bodies are more vulnerable to toxins.

THIMEROSAL

Thimerosal is a mercury-based preservative in some vaccines to prevent bacterial and fungal contamination. Mercury is a well-known neurotoxin that can cause severe damage to the nervous system. Despite assurances from health authorities that the levels of thimerosal in vaccines are safe, many studies have linked mercury exposure to developmental and neurological disorders, including autism.

In 1999, thimerosal was removed from most childhood vaccines in the United States as a precautionary measure. However, it is still used in some flu vaccines and vaccines administered in other countries. The ongoing use of thimerosal in vaccines continues to be a contentious issue, particularly among those concerned about its potential impact on children's health.

POLYSRBATE 80

Polysorbate 80 is an emulsifier used in vaccines to help mix ingredients that would separate. This chemical is known to cause allergic reactions in some individuals and has been linked to an increased risk of infertility and cancer in animal studies.

There is also evidence that polysorbate 80 can increase the permeability of the blood-brain barrier, potentially allowing other harmful substances in vaccines to enter the brain. This could have severe implications for neurological health, particularly in infants and young children.

ANIMAL CELL LINES

Several vaccines are developed using animal cell lines, including those derived from monkeys (Vero cells), dogs (MDCK cells), and chickens (chicken embryo cells). These cell lines are used to grow viruses for vaccines. Using animal cell lines raises ethical and health concerns, as they can contain residual animal DNA and proteins.

Injecting foreign animal DNA into the human body can cause immune reactions and genetic mutations. The long-term health effects of these residual animal components are poorly understood, and their use in vaccines remains controversial.

ACETONE

Acetone is a solvent used in some vaccine manufacturing processes. It is commonly found in household products such as nail polish remover and paint thinners. Acetone is a volatile organic compound that can cause respiratory irritation, headaches, and dizziness with prolonged exposure.

The presence of acetone in vaccines, even in small amounts, raises concerns about its potential impact on health, particularly in young children who are more susceptible to toxins.

E. COLI

Some vaccines are produced using recombinant DNA technology, involving E. coli bacteria to produce vaccine components. While the bacteria are killed during manufacturing, residual bacterial proteins and endotoxins can remain in the final product.

These residual components can trigger immune responses and potentially cause adverse reactions. The safety of using genetically modified bacteria in vaccine production is a subject of ongoing debate and research.

YEAST

Yeast is used to produce some vaccines, particularly recombinant DNA technology. While yeast is generally considered safe, some individuals may have allergies or sensitivities to yeast proteins, which can cause allergic reactions or other adverse effects.

The potential for yeast allergies raises questions about the safety of these vaccines for individuals with known sensitivities.

GLUTARALDEHYDE

Glutaraldehyde is a disinfectant and preservative used in some vaccines to inactivate viruses and bacteria. It is a potent chemical that, with prolonged exposure, can cause respiratory irritation, skin burns, and allergic reactions.

The use of glutaraldehyde in vaccines raises concerns about its potential toxicity, particularly when injected into the body. Its effects on developing children and the long-term health implications are poorly understood.

THE ISSUE OF INJECTION
One of the most concerning aspects of vaccines is that the ingredients are injected directly into the body's closed system, bypassing the digestive system's natural detoxification pathways. This makes it difficult, if not impossible, for the body to effectively detoxify these substances, leading to their accumulation and potential long-term health effects.

If a parent were to concoct a drink containing these same ingredients and give it to their child, they would likely be charged with attempted murder due to the toxic nature of the substances. Yet, it is considered acceptable for the medical profession to inject these ingredients into children under the guise of immunization. This double standard raises serious ethical and health concerns that deserve public attention and scrutiny.

SIDE EFFECTS LISTED IN VACCINE INSERTS
Vaccine inserts often contain a list of potential side effects, some of which are deeply concerning. These can include:
- Sudden Infant Death Syndrome (SIDS)
- Autism
- Diabetes
- Guillain-Barré Syndrome (GBS)
- Seizures
- Anaphylaxis

- Chronic Fatigue Syndrome
- Autoimmune disorders
- Allergic reactions
- Developmental delays
- Behavioral issues

It's important to note that while these side effects are listed, health authorities often downplay them. Many chronic illnesses are not officially attributed to vaccines, but there is growing evidence to suggest a potential link. This is a short list. Some inserts have almost an entire page of KNOWN adverse effects.

THE 13.1 WARNING

The 13.1 warning on vaccine inserts states that the vaccine has not been evaluated for its carcinogenic or mutagenic potential or impairment of fertility, but it has been quietly removed from many inserts. This removal raises significant concerns about transparency and the disclosure of potential vaccine risks.

By eliminating the 13.1 warning, vaccine manufacturers and health authorities effectively conceal that these products have not undergone comprehensive testing for some of the most severe long-term health risks. This lack of transparency undermines public trust and calls into question the safety assurances provided by the vaccine industry.

The presence of potentially harmful ingredients in vaccines is a significant cause for concern. While health authorities assure the public that these substances are present safely, the cumulative effects of multiple vaccines and other environmental exposures raise serious questions about their safety.

Parents and individuals deserve to be fully informed about vaccine ingredients and potential risks. The debate over vaccine safety is not just about science but also about transparency, informed consent, and the right to make decisions about one's health and that of one's children. The only way to know for sure that your child won't be the one having the side effects is to forego the risk altogether.

Chapter 57:

Uncovering SV40: The Simian Virus Presence in Vaccines

A less-discussed aspect of vaccine production involves the presence of simian viruses, particularly SV40, in certain formulations. This chapter explores the scientific evidence surrounding SV40 in vaccines, shedding light on its potential health implications, mainly its association with certain cancers.

DISCOVERY AND ORIGIN

SV40, a virus derived from the rhesus monkey, was first identified in polio vaccines produced in the 1960s. These vaccines, developed using simian cell lines, inadvertently introduced SV40 into human populations. Although initially unrecognized, subsequent research uncovered its presence, sparking investigations into its biological effects.

The presence of SV40 in polio vaccines led to widespread exposure among vaccine recipients. This exposure raised concerns due to SV40's known ability to infect human cells and induce cancer in laboratory settings. The transmission of SV40 through vaccination became a focal point of scrutiny, prompting efforts to mitigate its potential risks.

HEALTH IMPLICATIONS

Scientific studies have demonstrated a link between SV40 exposure and certain cancers, including mesothelioma and brain tumors. These findings have raised concerns about the long-term health effects of SV40 contamination in vaccines.

While the exact mechanisms by which SV40 contributes to cancer development remain under investigation, its presence in vaccines has raised legitimate scientific questions about vaccine safety.

Regulatory agencies have implemented measures to address SV40 contamination in vaccines, including guidelines for using non-simian cell lines in vaccine production. These measures aim to minimize the risk of accidental exposure to SV40 and other simian viruses, safeguarding public health. Ongoing surveillance efforts continue to monitor vaccine safety and detect any adverse effects associated with SV40 contamination.

PUBLIC AWARENESS AND ADVOCACY

Efforts to raise public awareness about SV40 and its potential health implications have been met with varying degrees of success. Advocates have called for greater transparency in vaccine production processes and increased scrutiny of vaccine safety. By raising awareness of the scientific evidence surrounding SV40, advocates aim to empower individuals to make informed decisions about vaccination.

The presence of SV40 in vaccines underscores the importance of rigorous scientific evaluation and regulatory oversight in vaccine development and production. The association between SV40 and certain cancers warrants further investigation. By staying informed about the scientific evidence surrounding SV40 and advocating for transparency in vaccine production, individuals can play a role in demanding valid informed consent with vaccines.

Chapter 58

The Gap Between Informed Consent and Vaccine Information Sheets

Informed consent is mandatory in ethical medical practice, serving as a cornerstone of patient autonomy and decision-making. Regulatory agencies emphasize the importance of providing individuals with comprehensive information about medical interventions, including vaccines, to enable them to make informed choices about their health. However, the vaccine information sheets handed to parents at well-visits fall short of meeting the criteria for informed consent. Let's explore the concept of informed consent defined by regulatory agencies and highlight the discrepancies between this ideal and the reality of vaccine information sheets.

UNDERSTANDING INFORMED CONSENT

Informed consent is when individuals are provided with relevant information about a medical intervention, including its purpose, risks, benefits, alternatives, and potential outcomes. This information enables individuals to make voluntary, informed decisions about accepting or declining the proposed intervention. Fundamental principles of informed consent include voluntariness, comprehension, and capacity, ensuring that individuals have the freedom to choose and understand the implications of their choices.

Regulatory agencies, such as the U.S. Food and Drug Administration (FDA) and the Centers for

Disease Control and Prevention (CDC), provide guidelines for informed consent in medical practice, including vaccination. These guidelines emphasize the importance of transparency, honesty, and respect for individual autonomy in the informed consent process. Healthcare providers are encouraged to communicate openly and honestly with patients and ensure they have the information they need to make informed decisions about vaccination.

DISCREPANCIES IN VACCINE INFORMATION SHEETS

Despite regulatory requirements for informed consent, the vaccine information sheets distributed to parents at well-visits often fail to provide comprehensive and unbiased information about vaccines. These sheets typically focus on the benefits of vaccination while downplaying or omitting information about potential risks and adverse reactions. Critical details, such as the ingredients of vaccines, their known side effects, and the limitations of vaccine safety data, are often overlooked or obscured.

Furthermore, vaccine information sheets may lack context or nuance, presenting vaccines as a one-size-fits-all solution without considering individual circumstances or preferences. This one-sided presentation of information undermines the principles of informed consent and deprives individuals of the opportunity to make fully informed decisions about vaccination.

CLOSING THE GAP

To bridge the gap between regulatory standards for informed consent and the reality of vaccine information sheets, healthcare providers must prioritize open and honest communication with patients. This includes providing balanced and comprehensive information about vaccines, including their potential risks and benefits, and handling any questions or concerns that patients may have. By empowering people to make informed choices about vaccination, healthcare providers can uphold the principles of informed consent and respect patient autonomy.

Informed consent is fundamental to ethical medical practice, ensuring individuals have the information they need to make voluntary and informed decisions about their health. While regulatory agencies emphasize the importance of informed consent in vaccination, the vaccine information sheets provided to parents at well-visits fall short of meeting these standards. By recognizing the discrepancies between regulatory standards and the reality of vaccine information sheets, healthcare providers can work to improve communication and empower patients to make truly informed decisions about vaccination.

Monetizing Misery

Chapter 59

Well-Child Visits: Vaccination Mandates and the Erosion of Informed Consent

Well-child visits, intended to monitor a child's growth and development, have increasingly become synonymous with vaccination appointments. While ostensibly aimed at promoting children's health, these visits often prioritize vaccination above all else, leaving little room for meaningful discussion or consideration of individual circumstances. This chapter examines the transformation of well-child visits into vaccination appointments and the challenges to informed consent that arise in this context.

WELL-CHILD VISITS HAVE BECOME VACCINE VISITS

In recent years, well-child visits have evolved into vaccination appointments, with healthcare providers focusing primarily on administering vaccines according to recommended schedules. The pressure to vaccinate is pervasive, with healthcare professionals frequently emphasizing the importance of adherence to vaccination guidelines and downplaying concerns or questions raised by parents.

REFUSAL AND COERCION

Parents who express hesitation or refusal regarding vaccination are often met with resistance and coercion from healthcare providers. Refusal paperwork, commonly presented as a legal requirement, may include incriminating language suggesting neglect or endangerment if vaccines are declined. This coercive tactic can intimidate parents into compliance, regardless of their concerns or objections.

INFORMED CONSENT AND THE RIGHT TO REFUSE

True informed consent requires freely accepting or declining medical interventions, including vaccination, based on comprehensive information and personal beliefs. However, the current landscape of well-child visits often fails to uphold this principle, as parents are pressured to comply with vaccination mandates without considering their rights or preferences.

LEGISLATIVE HURDLES AND MANDATORY VACCINATION

Legislation mandating vaccination for school entry has further complicated the issue of refusal at well-child visits. In many jurisdictions, exemptions for medical, religious, or philosophical reasons are increasingly difficult to obtain, effectively coercing parents into compliance with vaccination requirements or facing barriers to accessing public education.

PRESERVING INFORMED CONSENT AND PARENTAL RIGHTS

In the face of mounting pressure to vaccinate at well-child visits, it is essential to uphold the principles of informed consent and respect parental rights. Healthcare providers must engage in open and honest dialogue with parents, providing balanced information about vaccines and acknowledging their right to refuse based on personal beliefs or medical considerations.

Well-child visits have become indelibly linked with vaccination appointments, creating challenges to informed consent and parental autonomy. The use of coercion, refusal paperwork, and legislative mandates undermines parents' fundamental rights to make informed decisions about their children's healthcare. By advocating for transparency, respect for parental rights, and meaningful dialogue, we can strive to preserve the integrity of well-child visits and uphold the principles of informed consent in pediatric healthcare.

Monetizing Misery

Chapter 60

The Unseen Hand of Ignaz Semmelweis

INVISIBLE THREATS

In the mid-19th century, amidst the hallowed halls of Vienna General Hospital, a sinister presence lurked, unbeknownst to all who traversed its corridors. The hospital, a bastion of medical knowledge, concealed an invisible enemy that wreaked havoc amongst its patients—an enemy that no one could see, smell, or touch.

The hospital's maternity clinic was a particularly grim stage for this silent adversary. A condition known as childbed fever, or puerperal fever, held sway over new mothers. Its symptoms were nightmarish—a relentless fever, searing abdominal pain, and an inexorable descent into agony. Death was the inevitable conclusion for many, robbing infants of their mothers and families of their beloved kin.

Amidst the despair, a young Hungarian physician named Ignaz Semmelweis undertook a harrowing investigation. His quest to unravel the mystery behind the rampant childbed fever. Yet, the prevailing medical wisdom offered no solace. Theories abounded—lousy air and even an alignment of the planets were all implicated. But in the shadows, the true culprits remained concealed.

REVELATION IN THE MORGUE

Semmelweis's pursuit of the truth led him to a gruesome discovery in the hospital's morgue. An unsettling pattern emerged—autopsies performed by medical students were intertwined with the high mortality rate in the maternity clinic. He was confronted by the chilling realization that the medical staff themselves were unwittingly complicit in the spread of childbed fever.

CONTAMINATED HANDS: AN UNSEEN MENACE

Semmelweis delved deeper into the morbid riddle, scrutinizing every detail of the hospital's operations. And then, the breakthrough—his revelation was as simple as it was profound. The answer lay not in the stars or the air but in the contaminated hands of the doctors. The invisible culprits were minuscule particles, invisible to the naked eye, transmitted from cadavers to the women via the physicians' hands.

With this revelation came an inescapable truth—childbed fever was not an inevitable curse but a preventable calamity. Semmelweis embarked on a crusade to enforce handwashing with chlorine for all medical personnel, a practice now so elementary yet so revolutionary in its time. However, he faced not only his peers' obstinacy but also the medical establishment's hubris. His fellow physicians—mostly upper-class gentlemen—were insulted by the suggestion that their hands weren't clean. They also took a stance against the scientific basis of his Semmelweis' proposed "cadaverous particles," which did not agree with their theories of disease. Imagine not understanding the principle of cross-contamination, which is in essence, what Semmelweis was pointing out. His entire message was instead of going directly from having hands in a cadaver, physicians should wash and then go deliver babies. In other words, and pertinent to vaccines, you cannot inject dead cells into the living.

THE SEMMELWEIS EFFECT

Semmelweis's efforts, though noble, were met with resistance, ridicule, and ultimately tragedy. He became a pariah in the medical community, his pioneering work dismissed, and his mental health deteriorated. He died in a mental asylum, a victim of the ailment he had fought so tirelessly to combat.

THE LEGACY OF SEMMELWEIS: LESSONS UNLEARNED

The tragedy of Ignaz Semmelweis serves as a poignant reminder of the human tendency to overlook the obvious, to resist change, and to scorn those who dare challenge convention. His story, immortalized as the "Semmelweis Effect," reverberates through the annals of medical history. It is a testament to the difficulty of shattering entrenched beliefs and an enduring plea for the relentless pursuit of truth, no matter how unpalatable it may be.

By now it should be apparent why Semmelweis made it into the book, but for the sake of clarity, I will expound. The entrenched belief is that vaccines do more good than harm. The people that fight this narrative face militant opposition sometimes amid threats and hateful wishes. It can be hard to stand against the crashing tide that is the prevalent ways of the biomedical model. The mantra of which seems to be: solve everything with drugs and if there is a side effect, more drugs. The Semmelweis effect is precisely why advocates of medical freedom, and especially vaccine abolitionists, continue the fight even when it is wearisome. Most of us aren't getting paid, in fact, we are spending our own money to make sure that information is made available to people, no matter where they are in their search for information.

Make no mistake, change is still resisted and scorn is sill doled out to anyone that would dare to challenge the conventions of our time. If you haven't experienced this yet, stick around, and you will.

Chapter 61

Terrain Theory Reigns Supreme

In the realm of medical theory, where ideas are both the architects of health and the sentinels of disease, two titans clash. On one side stands the venerable Germ Theory, a colossus championed by top names like Louis Pasteur, armed with the conviction that pathogens, those nefarious invaders from the outside, are the prime culprits behind the world's afflictions. On the opposing flank, in more shadowed yet intriguing corridors of medical thought, lies Terrain Theory.

DUELING DOCTRINES: GERM VS. TERRAIN THEORY

Germ Theory, like a sword of Damocles, hangs over modern medicine. It decrees that the invaders, the microbe marauders—bacteria, viruses, fungi—are the harbingers of human maladies. In this dogma, the remedy lies in their annihilation, cleansing the world of these microscopic adversaries. Such is the creed that gave birth to vaccines, antibiotics, and the white-coated healers of the modern age.

Yet, beneath the surface, Terrain Theory lurks in the whispers of contrarian voices. This theory whispers that the battleground is not solely the external world but the terrain within us. The "terrain," our inner kingdom, wields its own scepter of influence over health and disease. It dares to suggest that a robust internal environment, fortified by nutrition, lifestyle, and balance, is the true guardian against maladies.

THE HEART OF TERRAIN THEORY

Herein lies the core tenet: the strength of our defenses, the resilience of our immune citadel, and the vitality of our internal equilibrium determine whether the marauders can breach our gates. Terrain Theory unfurls the tapestry of health that weaves nutrition, lifestyle, and the delicate balance of our inner ecosystem into the fabric of our well-being.

It posits that pathogens, those shadowy foes, may linger among us, coexisting without malevolence when the terrain stands as a fortress of vigor. Yet, should our inner dominion falter, should the balance waver, these invaders may seize an opportunity to wreak havoc. The terrain theory asserts that we have a modicum of control over our own well-being and that the outside world isn't dangerous to us so long as we are maintaining optimal health. Of course, this is not a popular way of looking at health in a world where reading ingredients shows a chemical cocktail infesting our food. Of course, it is far easier to dine on drive-thru food than tend gardens and animals and prepare better food at home to ensure necessary nutrients are building our cells instead of overloading our organs with the work of digesting food not meant for human consumption.

As with any intellectual feud, the battle rages on. Germ Theory's flag flies high in the domain of mainstream medicine, its edicts carving the path to diagnosis, treatment, and prevention. But Terrain Theory, though cast in the shade, endures as a beacon for those who seek a more holistic compass. They believe in prevention through lifestyle, nutrition, and cultivating an inner Eden.

The terrain is rife with controversy, and the boundaries of these medical realms are ever-shifting. Yet, the debate, the perpetual yin and yang of theories, adds depth to understanding disease and wellness. Within the tapestry of these theories, the enigmatic interplay of external invaders and internal resilience continues to unravel, captivating those who seek to fathom the intricate dance of health and disease.

Ultimately, whether one aligns with the established dogma of Germ Theory or treads the uncharted territories of Terrain Theory, the quest for health and the mysteries of the human body persist as an enthralling narrative. This story remains open to exploration and reinterpretation. Sadly, the terrain theory has opened up the medical freedom movement to other wolves which will be revealed in the next book.

Chapter 62

The Hidden Code: Viruses Engraved in Our DNA

In the intricate tapestry of our DNA, a mesmerizing exposé unfolds, casting aside conventional beliefs and inviting us into the cryptic realm where viruses and humanity share an astonishing connection. Here, we challenge the prevailing notion that viruses are solely external invaders, venturing instead into the tangled hub of our genetic script.

VIRUSES EMBEDDED WITHIN
There is a lot of virology research that doesn't get much airtime because the need for certain remedies would be obsolete if the research were acknowledged publicly. While this book isn't meant to turn into a medical or biological tome, certain topics being brought to light will help make later connections clearer. Everyone has the same access to information via the internet, and anyone leading widespread movements should be immersed in the research of the field they are trying to steer opinion in. The Medical Freedom Movement has seemed to pick up the easier flags which means that many followers are left in the dark. I am attempting to eliminate that folly.

Back to the information.

At the core of this extraordinary saga lies the concept of viral integration, a concept that redefines our perception of viruses as mere intruders. Rather than being passive victims of viral onslaught, we've unwittingly welcomed viral elements into our genetic code.

ARCHITECTS OF EVOLUTION: RETROVIRUSES

Retroviruses, a remarkable class of viral architects, take center stage in this genetic masterpiece. These cunning entities possess the extraordinary ability to inscribe their own genetic melodies directly into our DNA. Once this union occurs, the virus becomes a permanent resident, forever etched within the double helix of our genes. Carrie Arnold, in her essay "The Non-Human Living inside of You," states "Eight percent of our DNA consists of remnants of ancient viruses, and another 40 percent is made up of repetitive strings of genetic letters that is also thought to have a viral origin."

There is much more research about isolated virus code in our DNA that has been recognized as turning health conditions off and on in our body. The research has tracked specific viruses as being protective in utero. So, are viruses as scary as the mainstream media and public sources would have you believe?

SILENT INHABITANTS: DORMANT VIRUSES

Integrated retroviruses aren't dormant in the conventional sense. Instead, they assume a subtle existence, evading the attention of our vigilant immune defenses. They persist quietly, like enigmatic verses in an ancient volume, awaiting their moment.

The mystery within this viral narrative lies in the potential for activation. These integrated viral sequences remain latent, sometimes for generations, only to reawaken under specific circumstances. One such catalyst is their proximity to an active infection.

FROM DORMANCY TO DANCE: CHICKEN POX

Let us consider the chicken pox virus, a notorious character in the world of human viruses. During childhood, it often pays a visit, bestowing upon us an itchy tapestry of crimson spots. But the tale doesn't conclude there. After this initial encounter, the chicken pox virus withdraws, incorporating its genetic composition into our own.

SHINGLES: THE VIRAL ENCORE

The known natural "boost"-ing power (a form of inoculation) of adults caring for children with chicken pox kept subsequent infections at bay for most healthy adults. The advent and administration of the varicella vaccine has opened adults up for a more dangerous version of childhood chicken pox.

Years, sometimes decades later, when our immune system faces new challenges or falters with age, the dormant chicken pox virus may rouse from its slumber. It stirs from within, adopting a new identity known as shingles. The previous dormant virus returns with a vengeance, manifesting as agonizing skin rashes and nerve inflammation.

THE INNER TRIGGER: ENERGETIC ACTIVATION

What prompts this reawakening, this internal activation of a seemingly inactive virus? This remains a beguiling conundrum. Some propose a weakened immune system as a catalyst. In contrast, others posit that environmental factors, stress, or the energy associated with proximity to an active infection may hold the elusive key.

I bring this up to simply show that there is much unknown. Next, I want to look at the measles virus, as also much ignored. This information is incredibly well researched and hidden which is a travesty since the MMR vaccine is one of the known top issues in causing adverse effects.

Chapter 63

Measles Virus as a Cancer Protectorate

In the quest to unlock the mysteries of cancer and harness the body's natural defenses, scientists have turned their attention to the most unexpected of allies: the measles virus. Once primarily feared for its contagious nature and potential for outbreaks, the measles virus is now emerging as a potential protectorate against cancer, offering a fascinating avenue for future medical research and treatment.

THE MEASLES VIRUS: A HISTORICAL PERSPECTIVE

Before delving into its role as a cancer-fighting agent, it's essential to understand the measles virus itself. Measles is a viral infection that primarily affects children. While it can cause severe health complications, including pneumonia and encephalitis, it generally confers immunity once the infection has been overcome. That means, for most people, once they have experienced measles, they will not have it again. Keep this in mind. This characteristic piqued the curiosity of scientists investigating its potential in cancer research.

ONCOLYTIC VIRUSES

The concept of using viruses to combat cancer isn't new. In fact, it dates back over a century when physicians noticed that some cancer patients who contracted viral infections experienced temporary remissions. This observation led to the development of oncolytic virotherapy, a treatment strategy where viruses are utilized to discriminately infect and destroy cancer cells while sparing healthy tissues.

MEASLES VIRUS AND CANCER: A SURPRISING CONNECTION

One of the most intriguing findings in recent years has been the link between the measles virus and its ability to target cancer cells. Research has shown that the measles virus exhibits a remarkable affinity for certain cancer cells. When introduced into a tumor, the virus selectively infects and destroys the malignant cells, leaving the surrounding healthy tissue unharmed.

THE MECHANISM BEHIND THE ANTI-CANCER ACTION OF MEASLES

Several mechanisms underpin the measles virus's anticancer properties:

1. Receptor Expression: Cancer cells often express specific surface receptors that make them vulnerable to viral infections. The measles virus is known to target and enter cells through the CD46 receptor, which is frequently overexpressed on the surface of cancer cells (Smith, Janessa).

2. Immunomodulation: Measles infection can stimulate the body's immune response, crucial for identifying and eliminating cancer cells. It appears to "wake up" the immune system, making it more vigilant in its surveillance against malignant cells.

3. Apoptosis Induction: Measles infection can trigger apoptosis, a process of programmed cell death, in cancer cells. This programmed self-destruction is essential for removing damaged or malignant cells from the body.

CLINICAL TRIALS AND POTENTIAL APPLICATIONS

The promising preclinical studies have paved the way for clinical trials exploring the use of the measles virus in cancer therapy. These trials investigate the virus's efficacy against various types of cancer, including ovarian, lung, and brain cancers.

Preliminary results have been encouraging, with some patients experiencing significant tumor reduction and prolonged survival. The measles virus is also being explored with other treatments like chemotherapy and immunotherapy to enhance its anticancer effects.

While the potential of the measles virus in cancer treatment is exciting, several challenges remain. These include optimizing the virus's delivery to tumors, minimizing side effects, and ensuring the virus does not harm healthy cells.

Furthermore, there is ongoing research into the genetic modification of the measles virus to enhance its anticancer properties.

Using the measles virus as a protectorate against cancer represents a remarkable fusion of historical insights and cutting-edge science. As research advances, there is genuine hope that the once-feared measles virus could become a potent weapon in our arsenal against one of humanity's most relentless foes - cancer.

This leads to questions in my mind: Why does the Medical Freedom Movement call for safer vaccines when we know that immunity exists after only a week of sickness. Natural immunity seems far superior to risking adverse events. Furthermore, why are some of the Medical Freedom Movement leaders holding patents or have done research on single vaccines for the measles and other viruses? This seems counterintuitive to me.

SECTION EIGHT:

My Contributions to the Fight

Chapter 64

Handing Out My "Are Vaccines Safe?" Truth Cards

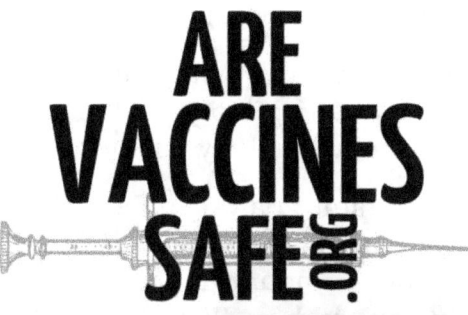

In addition to:

> ➢ my nonstop work to awaken the masses to the dangers of vaccines before, during, and since VaxXed came out,
>
> ➢ promoting VaxXed,
>
> ➢ hoping and praying while I spent numerous hours a day online advocating for children and awareness,

- believing that this group of 'characters' would have the impact needed to get changes made as they promised,
- to building a massive website (www.gregwyatt.com) containing information on the Health Freedom Movement, vaccines, etc,
- writing books to combat eugenics and tell-al about the history that has been forced upon me and my family;

Part of my relentless pursuit to awaken people to the risks of unthinkingly administering vaccines to their babies, I was driven by the haunting memory of the suffering endured by my children, Weston and Emily. Their plight served as a constant reminder of the hidden dangers lurking within those seemingly innocuous shots.

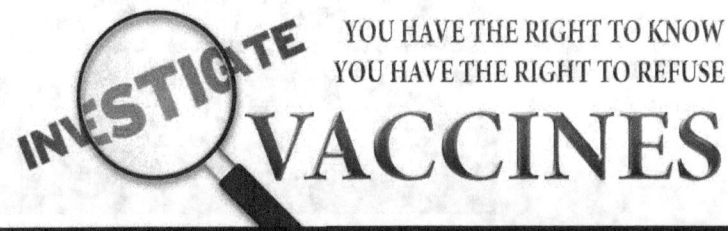

Armed with this fervent conviction, I set out to create a tool for enlightenment. Designing my logo and crafting informational cards, I awaited their arrival eagerly. When the box finally arrived in early 2016, containing the fruits of my labor, a wave of emotions washed over me.

> **IMPORTANT FACTS TO CONSIDER**
>
> ***Vaccines are not tested against true inert placebos.***
> If a vaccine injures, disables or kills you - you cannot sue the maker.
> *Some vaccines only protect recipient, do not contribute to "herd immunity"*
> ALL vaccines wear off over time - ALL vaccines can fail to protect
> *The current childhood schedule hasn't been tested for cumulative effects*
> Vaccines have not been tested for carcinogenic/mutagenic potential or to determine risks to unborn fetus before recommending during pregnancy.
> **ALL VACCINES HARM - VACCINE INJURIES ARE NOT RARE**
>
> **AreVaccinesSafe.org**

With the cards in hand, my next challenge lay distributing them effectively. Recognizing the power of personal interaction, I resolved to engage directly with parents needing enlightenment. Nervously at first but with growing confidence, I approached young mothers in supermarkets and other locations frequented by families.

My efforts soon expanded beyond personal outreach. I recruited fellow mothers from supermarkets, parks, and from the streets in Arizona, offering them a small stipend to distribute cards and gather statistics. Together, we blanketed our community with information, strategically placing cards in areas where parents were most likely to encounter them.

Despite resistance from pro-vaccine advocates, I persisted in my mission, undeterred by the challenges. Harnessing the power of social media, I shared the harrowing story of my vaccine-injured children with audiences around the world, dedicating countless hours to spreading awareness.

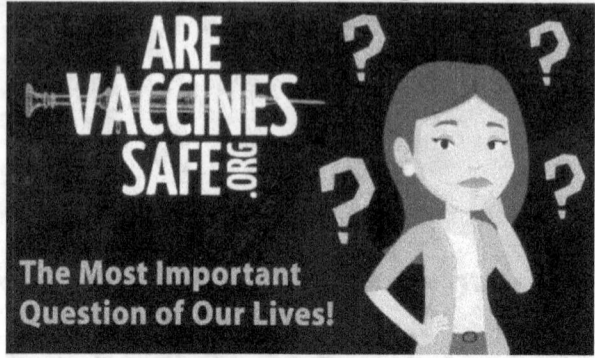

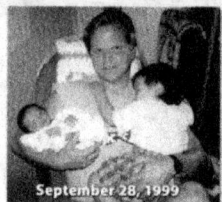

My son Weston was born on Groundhog's Day, Feb. 2nd, 1998; and his sister Emily was born on Sept. 14th, 1999. Both were born PERFECT with ZERO issues! Both suffered permanent and irreversible neurological damage from childhood vaccinations.

Weston is now 23 and intellectually functions at a 3-4 year old level and is deaf. Emily is now 21 and functions at a 7-8 year old level. Both require 24/7 care... and will for the rest of their lives.

Please **INVESTIGATE BEFORE YOU VACCINATE!** **Don't** listen to doctors and governments who make **BILLIONS** telling you *"vaccines are safe and effective!"* **Visit AreVaccinesSafe.org and ShotsOfTruth.com and discover the facts!**

This endeavor became more than just a passion project—a full-time commitment. Day in and day out, I devoted myself to the cause, driven by the belief that every card handed out was a potential life saved. I refused to monetize the pain of others, finding solace in the knowledge that my efforts were making a difference.

As I look at my kids every day, I promise myself to help educate families about vaccines, to save another family from going through a lifetime of struggles, and to make this world a better place. I just want to help create a safer, more informed world.

VACCINE INJURY MEMORIAL VEHICLE

Each day, I wake up renewed to continue this battle as long as God allows and provides.

Each day, I load up with as many cards as I can, put them in my pockets, hop in my vaccine injury memorial vehicle, and hit the streets and highways of Arizona. Things have changed a lot in the last seven years since I started doing this. People are much more open since the COVID fiasco as they realize all their friends have died and got injured from the jabs. Seven years ago, people would give me a little blowback daily. Now, all I get is honking horns, thumbs up, and positive affirmations as people realize the truth. I am happy that I was a part of it.

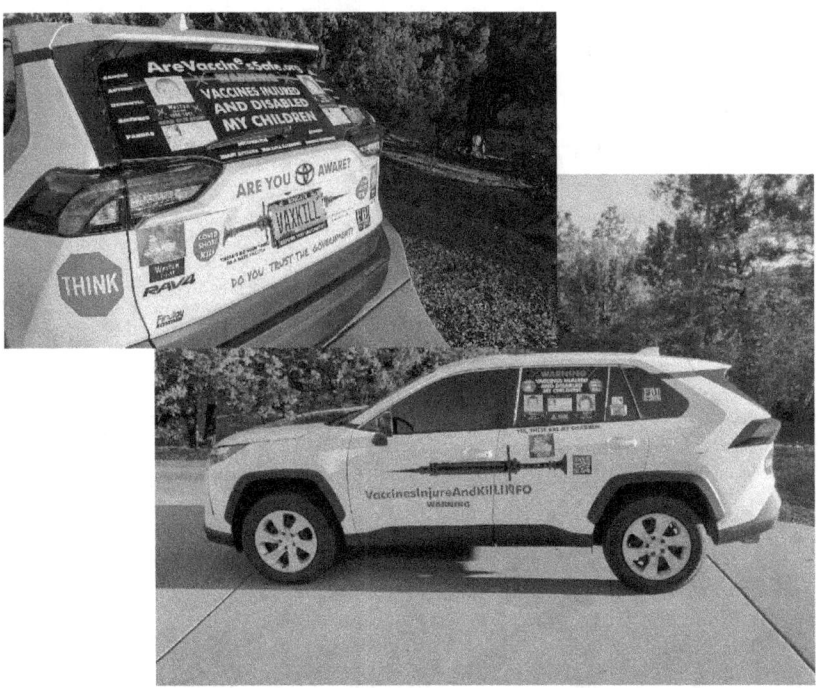

Monetizing Misery

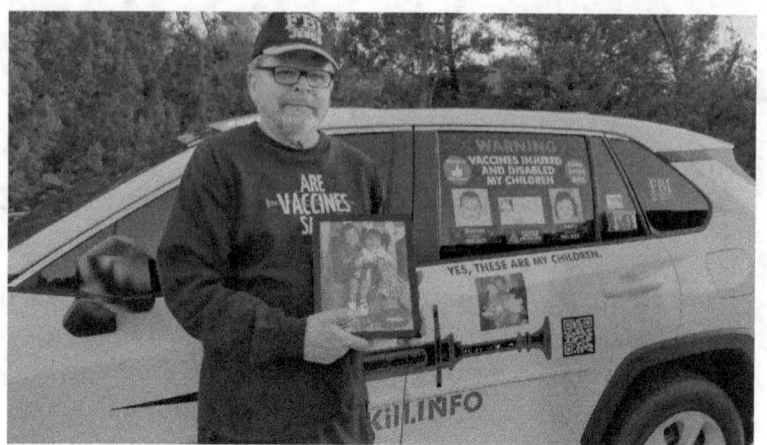

Chapter 65

The Weaponization of Social Media: Censorship, Propaganda, and Controlling the Narrative

To engage people who haven't heard the dangers of vaccines or the stories of parents who have already lived through the devastating effects of vaccine damage in their children, there has to be a platform for our voices to be heard.

Many of you have connected with my social media presence. Social media has created many frustrating moments for me over the years. I have had YouTube channels shut down as they reached millions with the story of Weston and Emily. Building the different audiences, I enjoy interacting with, took a lot of effort.

Watching them dissolve into thin air with my content with no warning was like taking a punch to the face and gut simultaneously. The frustration was palpable, draining the fight out of me; I entertained the thought of giving up. My profiles have spent time in social media "jails" where I was unable to interact with followers, correct false narratives that were being presented on my posts, and my voice was stopped much like it would have been in a book-burning Germany or a Communist country. Since we have to navigate these platforms to share our stories and collective knowledge, I want to dive deep into the censorship machine that social media has created and explain why it has been done this way.

THE RISE OF SOCIAL MEDIA CONTROL

In 2006, with the emergence of platforms like MySpace then Facebook, followed by the plethora of sites available now, the communication landscape underwent a profound transformation. What began as a means of connecting individuals has since evolved into a formidable force in shaping global narratives: social media. Over the years, this digital realm has expanded into a vast metaverse, increasingly dominated by major corporations with far-reaching vested interests. Among these interests are ties to pharmaceutical giants and other influential entities, underscoring the complex interplay between social media and corporate power.

This chapter explores the transformative impact of social media on public discourse, particularly in light of the COVID-19 pandemic. As the world grappled with unprecedented challenges, social media emerged as both a battleground for ideas and a conduit for control. From the suppression of dissenting voices under the guise of combating misinformation to the propagation of propaganda tailored to manipulate public opinion, the pandemic laid bare the immense power wielded by those who control the digital narrative.

I will shed light on the complicated dynamics at play by examining censorship, political silencing, and the exploitation of social media for propagandistic ends. As we delve into the intricacies of social media's influence, it becomes increasingly apparent that the metaverse is not merely a neutral space for exchange but a relatively contested terrain where competing interests vie for dominance and where big corporations have paid to play—to silence anyone who could cause their profit margins damage—even if the damage were caused by the truth (which is often the case).

In confronting the challenges posed by social media control, we must consider fundamental questions about the nature of democracy, the role of corporate influence, and the future of public discourse. We can work towards a digital landscape that upholds transparency, accountability, and freedom of expression by critically engaging with these issues. As we embark on this exploration, let us navigate social media's complexities with clarity, courage, and a steadfast commitment to the values underpinning our democratic societies.

PANDEMIC PARADIGM: A PREFACE TO EXTREME CENSORSHIP

The outbreak of the COVID-19 pandemic marked a turning point in the evolution of social media censorship. Censorship always existed for those of us within the anti-vax and "Health Freedom Movement." The powers that be (the decision makers) found the message of proper informed consent and the ability to make medical decisions for oneself very "dangerous." Nothing we presented was ever in opposition to the law--in fact, we were asking for the law to be upheld (informed consent, etc.).

As the world grappled with the unprecedented challenges posed by the virus, social media platforms became battlegrounds for competing narratives and information dissemination. However, what emerged was not merely a clash of ideas but a concerted effort by platform operators to curb the spread of what they deemed to be misinformation.

Social media companies implemented stringent censorship measures under the pretext of safeguarding public health and combating the dissemination of false or misleading information. Voices dissenting from official narratives or presenting alternative viewpoints became increasingly marginalized and silenced. Whether it was questioning the efficacy of particular public health measures, challenging the virus's origin, or advocating for alternative treatments, individuals and groups encountered swift and decisive censorship.

Crucially, the criteria for determining what constituted misinformation often remained opaque and subject to interpretation by platform moderators. This lack of transparency intensified concerns about the arbitrary nature of censorship and its potential to stifle legitimate debate and dissent. As a result, individuals who sought to engage in nuanced discussions or express skepticism towards prevailing narratives found themselves met with censorship rather than open dialogue.

The consequences of this censorship extended beyond the suppression of individual voices to encompass broader implications for democratic discourse. In a functioning democracy, the free exchange of ideas and perspectives is essential for informed decision-making and public accountability. However, censorship on social media platforms threatened to undermine these foundational principles, erecting barriers to the free flow of information and impeding the public's ability to evaluate and engage with complex issues critically.

The pandemic paradigm underscored the challenges inherent in navigating the tension between public health imperatives and civil liberties. While there is undoubtedly a need to combat the spread of misinformation that poses genuine risks to public health, the blanket suppression of dissenting voices raises troubling questions about the erosion of fundamental rights and freedoms in the digital age.

In confronting the pandemic paradigm of censorship on social media platforms, we have an obligation to strike a delicate balance between safeguarding public health and upholding democratic principles. This requires greater transparency in the decision-making processes of platform operators, robust mechanisms for appealing censorship decisions, and a commitment to fostering open and inclusive dialogue on matters of public concern. Only through such measures can we mitigate the chilling effects of censorship and preserve the integrity of democratic discourse in the digital era.

"POLITICAL" SILENCING: THE TYRANNY OF "MAJORITY" OPINION—PERCEIVED OR REAL, WE'LL NEVER KNOW

Beyond public health discourse, social media platforms have increasingly become arenas for suppressing political dissent. In a democratic society, the free exchange of ideas and perspectives is vital for fostering a vibrant public discourse and holding those in power accountable. However, the rise of social media censorship has led to the marginalization and silencing of voices that challenge mainstream ideologies or critique governmental policies.

At the heart of this phenomenon lies the "tyranny of majority opinion," wherein dominant societal narratives and prevailing political ideologies dictate the boundaries of acceptable discourse. Those who deviate from these norms often find themselves subjected to censorship, de-platforming, or other forms of digital suppression. In effect, social media platforms have become echo chambers where dissenting voices are systematically excluded, hindering the possibility of genuine dialogue and democratic deliberation.

The consequences of political silencing extend far beyond the individual level to encompass broader implications for democratic governance. When certain perspectives are suppressed or marginalized, the marketplace of ideas becomes impoverished, depriving society of diverse viewpoints and alternative solutions to pressing social and political issues. Moreover, the suppression of dissenting voices undermines the principles of pluralism and tolerance, essential components of any healthy democracy.

One of the most insidious aspects of political silencing on social media is its disproportionate impact on marginalized communities and historically oppressed groups. Minority perspectives that challenge entrenched power structures or advocate for social justice often face heightened levels of censorship and digital suppression. This perpetuates existing inequalities and reinforces patterns of marginalization, further entrenching the status quo.

Political silencing raises profound questions about the role and responsibilities of social media platforms in a democratic society. As private entities with significant influence over public discourse, these platforms wield considerable power in shaping political narratives and influencing public opinion. However, their exercise of this power could be more transparent and accountable, leading to concerns about censorship and bias.

In confronting the challenge of political silencing on social media, it is essential to reaffirm the principles of free speech, pluralism, and participation. This requires greater transparency and accountability from platform operators and the development of robust mechanisms for protecting political dissent and ensuring the diversity of voices in the digital public square. By fostering an environment that values open dialogue and respects the rights of all citizens to participate in the political process, we can safeguard the integrity of democratic governance in the digital age.

The problem isn't just that WE are silenced...the problem is that we have NO idea HOW MANY messages and how much information is missing from our discussions because someone somewhere decided that the people don't have their permissions or the right to free speech or the access to what others are exercising their free speech on. If you don't see the problem there, I can't help you.

THE EASE OF PROPAGANDA DISSEMINATION

The architecture of social media platforms inherently lends itself to the rapid spreading of propaganda, enabling manipulative actors to exert significant influence over public opinion on a global scale. Unlike traditional media channels, which are subject to editorial oversight and fact-checking processes, social media offers a decentralized and largely unregulated environment where misinformation and propaganda can flourish unchecked.

Central to the ease of propaganda dissemination on social media is the viral nature of content sharing. Algorithms prioritize engagement metrics such as likes, shares, and comments, incentivizing the production and expansion of sensationalist or emotionally charged content. This creates a fertile ground for propagandists to exploit, as provocative or misleading narratives are more likely to gain traction and reach a broad audience.

The targeting capabilities of social media advertising enable propagandists to tailor their messaging to specific demographics or interest groups, further enhancing the effectiveness of their campaigns. By leveraging data analytics and user profiling techniques, propagandists can identify vulnerable populations and deliver tailored content to elicit desired responses or manipulate perceptions.

The phenomenon of echo chambers aggravates the problem of propaganda dissemination on social media. As users curate their online experiences to align with their existing beliefs and preferences, they are more susceptible to confirmation bias and selective exposure to information. This creates fertile ground for propagandists to exploit, as individuals within echo chambers are less likely to evaluate or fact-check the content they encounter critically. The "fact-checkers" used on most social media platforms are hired and maintained by the liberal left, which may benefit your ideologies if that is the side you're on, but it can be most unfortunate if the truth is what is being sought. Many people have concluded that you can trust the information within the post if there is a "fact-check" on a post. Part of this distrust of social media is not just their sins of omission (our voices) but their sins of commission (the things they do allow on their platforms.

The anonymity afforded by social media platforms enables propagandists to operate with impunity, shielding their identities and motives from scrutiny. This lack of accountability further complicates efforts to combat propaganda and misinformation, allowing bad actors to evade detection and evade consequences for their actions.

In confronting the challenge of propaganda dissemination on social media, addressing the underlying structural vulnerabilities that enable its spread is essential. This requires greater transparency and accountability from platform operators and the development of robust mechanisms for detecting and mitigating the impact of propaganda campaigns. Additionally, efforts to promote media literacy and critical thinking skills among users are essential for protecting against the influence of propaganda and fostering a more resilient digital public sphere. By collectively addressing these challenges, we can work towards a social media ecosystem that is more resistant to manipulation and conducive to informed public discourse.

Chapter 66

Corporate Influence and Political Agendas

Social media platforms have become fertile ground for corporations and special interest groups to advance their agendas and influence public opinion. With the ability to target specific demographics and personalize content, these entities can leverage social media to shape narratives, promote products, and sway political discourse.

Corporations and special interest groups utilize various tactics to influence social media platforms. One prevalent strategy is paid promotions and sponsored content, where organizations pay to amplify their messages to a broader audience. These entities can effectively control the narrative and shape public perception by investing significant resources into targeted advertising campaigns.

There needs to be more clarity between genuine discourse and commercial interests to maintain journalistic integrity. Traditional media outlets, facing competition from social media platforms, may succumb to the pressures of sensationalism or bias to attract viewership and advertising revenue. This erosion of journalistic standards further amplifies the influence of corporate interests on public discourse, undermining the credibility of media institutions and distorting the flow of information.

The intersection of big tech and big pharma has raised concerns about the influence of corporate interests on public health discourse. Allegations of collusion between social media giants and pharmaceutical companies, particularly during health crises like the COVID-19 pandemic, highlight the potential for corporate agendas to shape public policy and perception. The proliferation of sponsored content and targeted advertising by pharmaceutical companies further complicates efforts to discern the truth and navigate complex health-related issues.

The pervasive influence of corporate interests on social media platforms underscores the need for greater transparency and accountability in digital communication. Efforts to mitigate the impact of corporate influence must include measures to increase transparency around sponsored content and targeted advertising and strengthen regulations governing political advertising and corporate lobbying efforts.

Raising media literacy and critical thinking skills among social media users is essential for inoculating against the influence of corporate propaganda and misinformation. By empowering individuals to critically evaluate the content they encounter and discern fact from fiction, we can build a more resilient digital public sphere that is less susceptible to manipulation by corporate interests.

In confronting the challenge of corporate influence on social media, it is imperative to uphold principles of transparency, accountability, and democratic participation. By promoting greater transparency in digital communication and fostering a culture of critical inquiry and media literacy, we can mitigate the influence of corporate agendas and ensure that the digital public sphere remains a space for open and informed discourse.

FROM MYSPACE TO METAVERSE: CONSOLIDATING CONTROL

The evolution of social media platforms from the early days of MySpace to the present-day metaverse has witnessed a significant consolidation of control in the hands of a select few corporate entities. What began as decentralized platforms for user-generated content has morphed into a digital landscape dominated by tech giants with unparalleled influence over global communication and discourse.

One of the defining features of this consolidation of control is the centralization of user data and content within a handful of platforms. Social media companies collect vast amounts of data on user behavior, preferences, and interactions, which they leverage to optimize engagement, target advertising, and shape the user experience. This centralized control over user data grants these platforms unprecedented power to influence the flow of information and shape public opinion.

The emergence of the metaverse—a virtual reality space where individuals can interact with digital environments and each other—represents a new frontier in consolidating control. Tech giants are vying to establish dominance in this emerging market, leveraging their resources and infrastructure to shape the development of the metaverse according to their interests and agendas.

The consequences of this consolidation of control are profound, with implications for the ability of individuals to freely express themselves and access diverse viewpoints. As social media platforms increasingly algorithmically curate content to maximize engagement and profitability, there is a risk of creating echo chambers where users are exposed only to information that reinforces their beliefs and perspectives.

Centralizing control within a few corporate entities raises concerns about transparency, accountability, and the concentration of power. With tech giants wielding unprecedented influence over public discourse and communication, there is a risk of these platforms being used to promote narrow interests, suppress dissent, and manipulate public opinion. The only thing we can do is keep showing up. There have been many days when I wanted to throw in the towel, hang up my hat, and after taking a breather away from the platform, I was able to clear my head and come back.

Greater regulatory oversight and accountability mechanisms are needed to curb the unchecked power of tech giants and ensure that the digital public sphere remains a space for open and inclusive discourse. A larger problem looms, the problem of big tech and big pharma linking arms, and we will deal with it in the next chaper.

Chapter 67

The Intersection of Big Tech and Big Pharma

Allegations of collusion between social media giants and pharmaceutical companies have emerged, particularly during health crises such as the COVID-19 pandemic. This intersection of big tech and big pharma raises significant concerns about the potential influence of corporate interests on public health discourse and policymaking through controlled narratives on social media. We know they colluded because within minutes of expressing concerns or issues with the vaccine, censorship started. There were people spending half their time unable to use social media platforms as more than a mere viewing device.

During the COVID-19 pandemic, social media platforms were central in spreading information about the virus, its transmission, and potential treatments. However, alongside legitimate public health messaging, there were widespread reports of misinformation, conspiracy theories, and promotional content from pharmaceutical companies seeking to capitalize on the crisis. And yes, the Health Freedom Movement became extremely lucrative during the pandemic.

Pharmaceutical companies have turned to social media platforms to promote their products, target specific demographics, and shape public perception. These companies seek to influence consumer behavior and drive demand for their products through sponsored content, targeted advertising, and influencer partnerships.

The potential influence of big pharma on social media extends beyond advertising to include the dissemination of medical information and the shaping of public health narratives. Reaching millions of users instantaneously, social media platforms have become powerful tools for amplifying pharmaceutical messaging and shaping public opinion on health-related issues.

The close relationship between big tech and big pharma raises concerns about conflicts of interest, transparency, and accountability. As social media companies increasingly rely on advertising revenue from pharmaceutical companies, there is a risk of prioritizing commercial interests over public health considerations.

The implications of this intersection extend beyond the realm of public health to encompass broader issues of corporate influence, regulatory capture, and democratic governance. With social media platforms playing an increasingly central role in shaping public discourse and opinion, it is essential to scrutinize the relationships between tech giants and pharmaceutical companies and ensure that they are not unduly influencing public health policy or eroding trust in scientific expertise.

In confronting the challenge of the intersection of big tech and big pharma on social media, there isn't an immediate solution. Money seems to have become far more important than human life. It seems the money collectors have forgotten that it takes human hands to exchange such money, so maybe they should protect life again. Efforts to strengthen regulations governing pharmaceutical advertising, increase transparency around sponsored content, and promote independent scientific research are essential for safeguarding public health and ensuring that social media platforms serve the public interest rather than narrow corporate agendas. The problem is Health Freedom Movement groups come in to monetize misery on the other side, peddling snake oils and bottling fear in a different container.

Monetizing Misery

Epilogue:
A Call to Awareness and Action

This book is not a comprehensive examination of the complex and multifaceted issues surrounding vaccines, eugenics, and the agenda to confuse and destroy. While we have delved into various aspects of these topics, significant areas remain unexplored within these pages. Institutions such as the CDC and FDA play pivotal roles in the vaccine narrative and are not extensively covered here. There are entire books dedicated solely to these agencies, and without expanding this work into tens of thousands of pages, it would be impossible to do justice to the depth and breadth of their influence and operations.

We have touched on the sinister workings of the pharmaceutical cartel and their modus operandi. However, rather than attempting to connect countless events and create an exhaustive timeline, the focus has been on illustrating the overarching mechanisms of control and manipulation. The pharmaceutical industry operates like an organized crime syndicate, with tactics and strategies that mirror the mob. This approach allows us to understand the fundamental nature of their operations without getting lost in the minutiae of endless events and scandals.

The lives affected and destroyed by this ever-evolving agenda are countless, and their stories deserve to be told. This book aims to shed light on how public health, personal autonomy, and informed consent are undermined. However, it is essential to acknowledge that covering every nuance and emerging development is a Herculean task. New information and revelations come to light daily, adding another layer to the complex narrative.

In closing, this book is a call to awareness and action. It is an invitation to question, research, and critically examine the information presented by those in positions of power. While this work provides a snapshot of the larger picture, it is up to each of us to continue seeking the truth and advocating for transparency, accountability, and the preservation of personal freedom. Our advocacy for these principles is not just a choice, but a responsibility that we all share. The journey towards understanding and exposing the full extent of the vaccine agenda is ongoing, and together, we can strive to protect future generations from the harms that have befallen so many.

Thank you for joining me in this exploration. Stay vigilant, stay informed, and never stop questioning. The fight for truth and justice is far from over.

A Letter from a Parent:

Here is a message I received from a parent who was also interviewed by VaxXed and didn't have such a great experience:

Dear Greg,

This is my experience with VaxXed along with many others.

It was the fall of 2016 and we were like thousands of others so excited to go meet the VaxXed bus it was fall of 2016.

This was our experience. First, the people there were not overly friendly. Everyone was cold and in a hurry. It was like we were just a number in a production and we were not the only ones that picked up on it. Call it a gut feeling but I expected more embracing, emotionally. Then Polly came bee bopping out of the bus and ushered us in.

Greg, I had spent hours getting her old medical records together, finding the pages where it stated that my daughter is never to have a DPT shot again, photocopied them, then laminated them so I could show them around forever without fear of them getting torn or stained. She never bothered to look at them and I think my daughter and I made history as the shortest interview EVER. It was about 5 minutes. We had driven hours and hours. Then she looked my daughter in the eyes and said " We are going to get you out of that group home and into a place you will love (THE AUTISM TRUST) and that was it.

So what's up telling us and countless others that? How cruel! Just because my precious daughter is brain-injured, doesn't make her stupid! Good thing she didn't put much weight into that comment! Face it, false hopes is what they sell while collecting and raising money for a project that does the way they explain it.

Within moments we were ushered out quickly and NO ONE asked me or anyone else for any contact info on. They just wanted us to sign "The VaxXed Bus" and send us on our way.

Polly told us and everyone else they had bought land in Texas and are building a huge community for the "special" folks BUT, some of them are families that signed over all of their assets.

At the time we or no one else had an idea that this was a business. A business of making money off the vaccine injured and dead.

I like many of my friends, want our name OFF that bus!

Feel free to repost this in hope that others can see the truth!

Sandy Lewis

References

(Ch. 27: Hollywood is THE Propaganda Machine)

    Redmond, Pearse. "The Historical Roots of CIA-Hollywood Propaganda." *The American Journal of Economics and Sociology*, vol. 76, no. 2, 2017, pp. 280–310. *JSTOR*, http://www.jstor.org/stable/45129369. Accessed 3 Sept. 2023.

(Chapter 31: Follow the Money – The Lucrative Pandemic-Fueled Windfall for Alleged 'Anti-Vaccination' Groups)

    Zadrozny, Brandy. *Once Struggling, Anti-Vaccination Groups Have Enjoyed a Pandemic Windfall*, www.nbcnews.com/tech/internet/struggling-anti-vaccination-groups-enjoyed-pandemic-windfall-rcna14402.

(Chapter 39: Collapsing Tragedy: The Untimely Death of Alex Spourdalakis)

    Ellis, Shân. "New Film Provides Insight into Life of a Mother Who Killed Autistic Son." *Autism Daily Newscast*, 25 Oct. 2016, www.autismdailynewscast.com/new-film-provides-insight-into-life-of-a-mother-who-killed-autistic-son/.

(Chapter 40: Capitalizing on Murder?: How Did They Miss the Warning Signs?)

    Joss, Laurel. "Documentary about Alex Spourdalakis Continues to Provoke Strong Reactions." Autism Daily Newscast, 8 Jan.

2015, www.autismdailynewscast.com/documentary-about-alex-spourdalakis-continues-to-provoke-strong-reactions/.

Picture credit: Blanco, Juan Ignacio. "Dorothy Spourdalakis: Photos: Murderpedia, the Encyclopedia of Murderers." *Dorothy Spourdalakis | Photos | Murderpedia, the Encyclopedia of Murderers*, murderpedia.org/female.S/s/spourdalakis-dorothy-photos.htm. Accessed 19 Jan. 2024.

(Ch. 47: SB277 - The Turning Point)

Pan, Richard. *SB-277 Public Health: Vaccinations.(2015-2016)*, leginfo.legislature.ca.gov/faces/billTextClient.xhtml?bill_id=201520160SB277. Accessed 11 Sept. 2023.

(Ch. 62: The Hidden Code: Viruses Engraved in Our DNA)

Arnold, Carrie. "The Non-Human Living inside of You." *Cold Spring Harbor Laboratory*, 15 Nov. 2022, www.cshl.edu/the-non-human-living-inside-of-you/.

(Ch. 63: Measles Virus as a Cancer Protectorate

Smith, Jenessa B., et al. "514. Targeting the Negative Immune Regulatory Molecule B7-H4 on Both Tumor and Normal Tissue With Anti-B7-H4 CAR T Cells." Molecular Therapy, 2015, https://doi.org/10.1016/s1525-0016(16)34123-5.

About the Author—Greg Wyatt

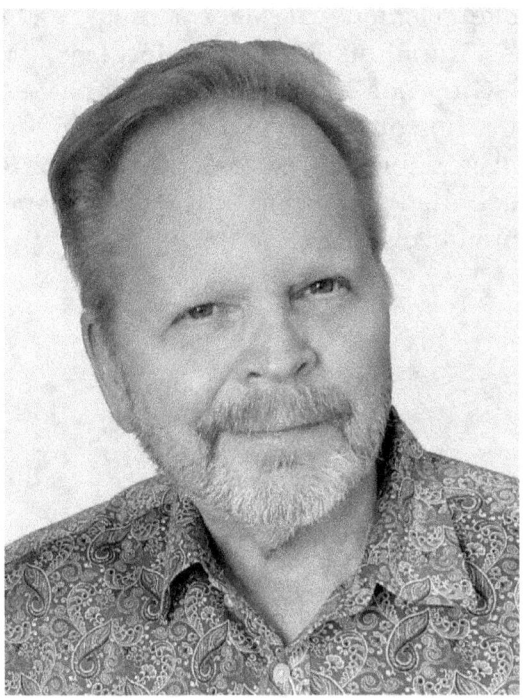

Greg Wyatt has dedicated his life to advocating for marginalized people and educating the public on critical issues that deeply impact our world. His personal experience of raising children with severe autism has only fueled his passion for shedding light on important topics.

Greg Wyatt has dedicated his life to advocating for the marginalized and educating the public on critical issues that profoundly impact our world. His personal experience of raising children with severe autism has only fueled his passion for shedding light on important topics such as autism, the dangers of vaccines, eugenics, and the exploitation of vulnerable populations.

Through his insightful and thought-provoking books like "Demons at My Doorstep," "Light in the Darkness," and his latest masterpiece, "Monetizing Misery," Greg has become a prominent voice to raise awareness on some of the most censored topics today. His tireless efforts to educate the public and bring positive change make him a beacon of hope for those facing similar challenges.

www.ingramcontent.com/pod-product-compliance
Lightning Source LLC
Chambersburg PA
CBHW071825210526
45479CB00001B/2